AF409347

INSIDE THIS ISSUE
STRENGTH TRAINING GUIDE FOR MENOPAUSAL WOMEN

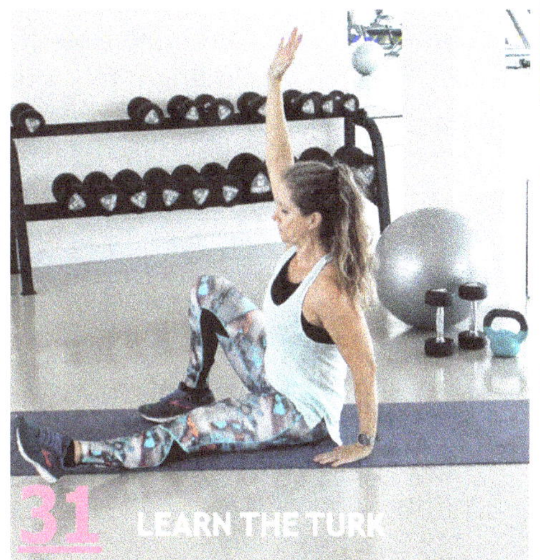

As we age, we need our muscles to be on point, as you would want to lift your bike into the car, bend over to tie your laces while running, go hiking or climb Kilimanjaro..

There is a very interesting study on why to what has motivated different women to compete or play sport. What is driving you? What motivates you?

The explanations and photos you are seeing in the document are all my own. No filters. You might see a wrinkle or two!

SIT: HIGH-INTENSITY SPRINT INTERVAL TRAINING

As a woman in her 40s, 50, 60s or above, we need to pay particular attention to how we train as athletes. The purpose of this guide is to provide some strength training that will serve you well as a menopausal athlete, as well as give you a little insight into our fabulous ageing bodies.

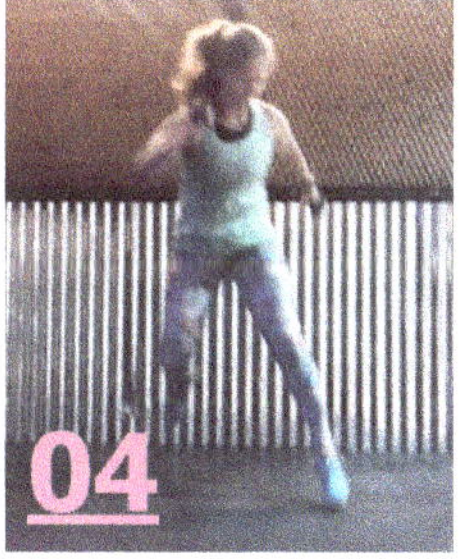

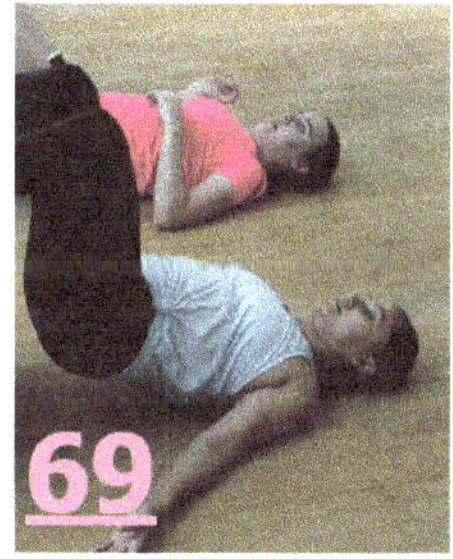

MENOPAUSE AND ME

I've exercised on and off my entire life. From a young age I was strongly encouraged to be slim...

RECOVERY

Without rest and proper recovery between workouts, your body will have difficulty when it comes to repair.

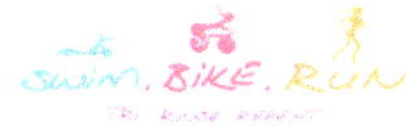

Contents

Disclaimer: this book has been written and published for informative purposes and should not be a substitute for actual instruction with a qualified person. The author is providing you with knowledge and information and how you choose to use that information is at your own risk. Please consult your sports doctor and/or physiotherapist before undertaking any exercise programme

ABOUT THE AUTHOR

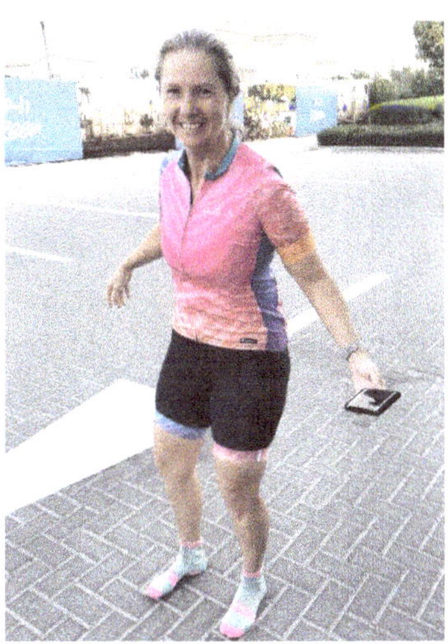 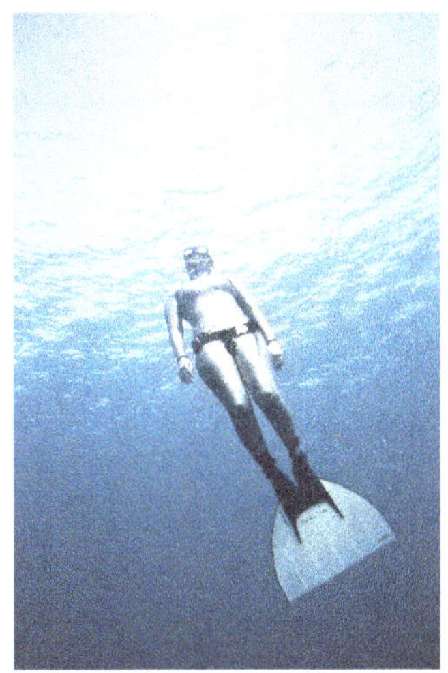 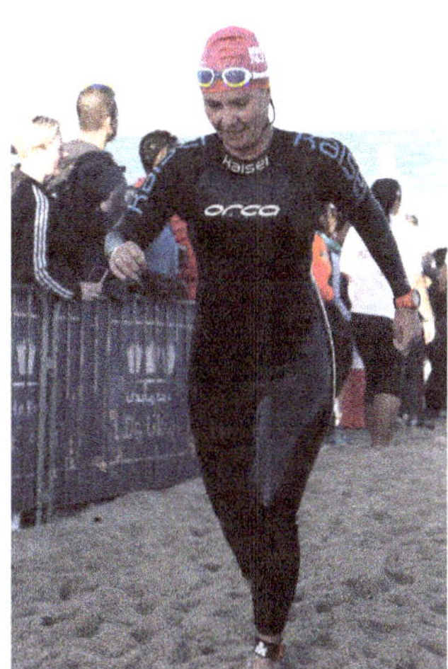

Sara Lise Harris is a sassy coach in her 50s who likes to approach training as a holistic journey to improve ability, agility and strength. Her aim is to improve performance, body relationships, and well-being in menopausal women.

A former Freediving and Scuba Diving Instructor for 22 years, she sought new challenges over the last decade and became an Ironman® Coach and Oceanman Open Water Swimming Coach in search of the ultimate way to find empowerment and strength in her athletic life. Importantly for this guide, she is also a certified NESTA kettlebell coach. She has practiced many different movements and programmes to help strengthen her own menopausal body to be able to continue participating in endurance sports and lead a fuller life.

MENOPAUSE AND ME

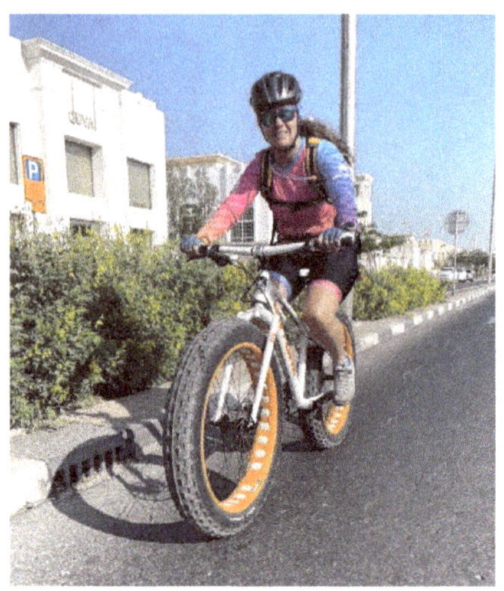

I've exercised most of my life. My parents were (are) very sporty and I was "encouraged", to be active and slim. Let's not go into the psychological aspects of this as this particular publication does not go that far, but I will say that there was a positive side to it in that I've always tried to stay fit and "normal bodied". Truth be told, I am a battler. The years of fad diets and yo-yo weight have had a negative effect on my endocrine system, resulting in hypothyroidism and adrenal insufficiency at the start of menopause. When my body started changing around the age of 46, training became physically and mentally difficult.

My waistline became squidgy, and it was really hard to get up in the mornings. My body grew increasingly puffier, I gained weight, felt a bit depressed and no matter how much "long slow distance" i did at the weekends, my body just grew. Outwards. My bits felt like they were Barbie's and occasionally like a doll I had when I was little (squeeze it and it pees, my body seemed to stink all the time (not sexy at all) and I just felt like I was ageing and rapidly!

A good friend Renette recommended a gynaecologist and she spoke to me at length about dietary changes, lifestyle changes (low carb diet (for a while), less alcohol (mostly), more sleep, (definitely) and also the benefits of taking Menopause Hormone Therapy. I also realised that I was going about my training in completely the wrong way. I started going to CrossFit (I was injured with tibial stress fracture and couldn't run), I did a Whole30 type regime for a few months and slowly introduced back some foods. I lost 10kgs and felt like a brand-new woman stepping out into a grey-haired menopausal planet with a new purpose.

MENOPAUSE AND YOU

As we age, we need our muscles to be on point, as you would want to lift your bike into the car, bend over to tie your laces while running, go hiking or climb Kilimanjaro, or even just enjoy an ocean swim without the sensation that your hamstrings have turned into piano wire. Whether you're in peri-menopause or over the other side like myself, a diet (not a fad diet, but balanced nutrition) and training interventions are super important to maintain strength, to maintain lean mass, bone support, posture, and prevent diseases such as diabetes and metabolic syndrome, even with exercise.

We need heavy strength and resistance training, plyometrics, SIT (high-intensity sprint interval training), as we are not only targeting the hypertrophy that occurs in muscle as we age, but the most important function:

- neuromuscular.

Menopausal women need to be gaining strength with the contraction of the muscle fibre, and not splitting their muscle fibre to make it bigger. I hear this often from women - "I don't want to lift weights as I will bulk out". You will not, if you do a combination of heavy resistance training plus some high- intensity training. This increases your post-exercise growth hormone, which again is a signal for tissue growth for developing lean mass and keeping it.

In many sport performances, the requirement is the ability to generate maximal muscular power, and this cannot be achieved by only running (for example).

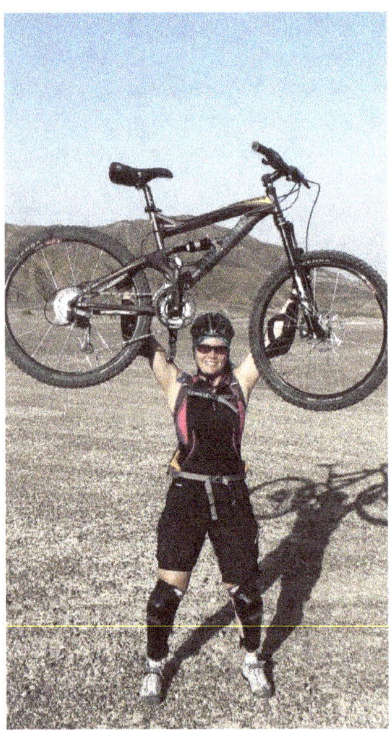

There is a very interesting study on why to what has motivated different women to compete or play sport. Sometimes the reasons are intrinsic, but often there are extrinsic reasons for participation.

The four extrinsic motivational regulations include:

1. External

2. Introjection

3. Identification

4. Integration

EXTERNAL regulation is the most highly controlled, or least autonomous, form of extrinsic motivation. It reflects behaviour stimulated by external stimuli, particularly the offering of rewards and/or threat of punishment.

INTROJECTED regulation, in contrast, is behaviour motivated by contingent consequences imposed by individuals on themselves.

IDENTIFIED regulation occurs when an individual accepts a behaviour's purpose or value as their own. That is, there is some degree of autonomy. Such as, an individual who exercises of their own volition because they believe in the health benefits brought about by exercise.

Lastly, **INTEGRATED** regulation represents the strongest form of internalized extrinsic motivation, where the individual not only endorses the purpose or value of the behaviour, but fully integrates it into his/her lifestyle and personality.

WHY STRENGTH?

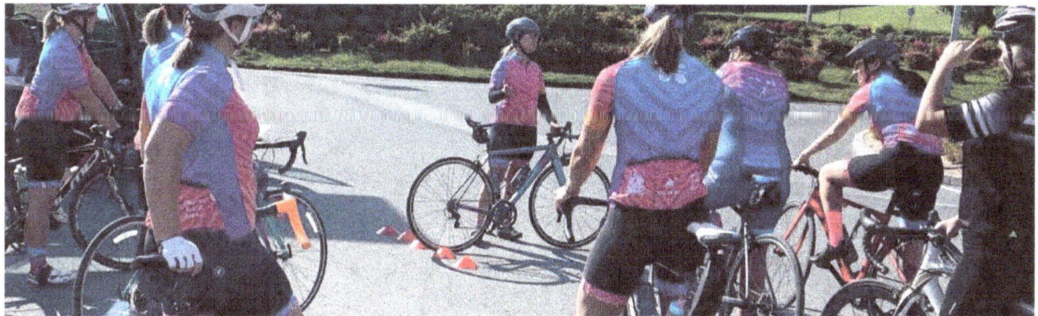

Every athlete needs to incorporate a strength training programme into their training, and it is essential for peri/menopausal women to do this, not only to become stronger and encourage lean muscle mass, but improved bone density to fight sarcopenia. Whatever your motivation is for doing this, a leisure pastime, or a personal challenge for something more competitive like age-grouping or getting to the World Championships, your strength journey should always be personal to you.

Whether you're training for a single sport or many, training can become boring or relentless, and coaches are keen to keep you interested and motivated to keep training. As a menopausal athlete, you (and your coach if you have one) need to understand the intricacies of your anatomy, physiology, mechanics, as programme design should apply these concepts as you are a unique individual. If you are reading this guide having downloaded a training plan of mine, you will need to consider the same elements. It takes significant time and effort to understand your athletic body.

Please read all the supplied articles and reference documents when you can as it could really help you achieve a more personalised experience and insight into all the research that has been done on menopausal women. Feelings of guilt or shame for missing a training session are examples of these contingent consequences. I have been guilty of this, and I have worked hard on giving myself permission to have a day off or two, because that's where the magic lies, in recovery!

You can contact me about my personalized programmes which can be done remotely, and my contact information is on the back cover.

IN THIS GUIDE

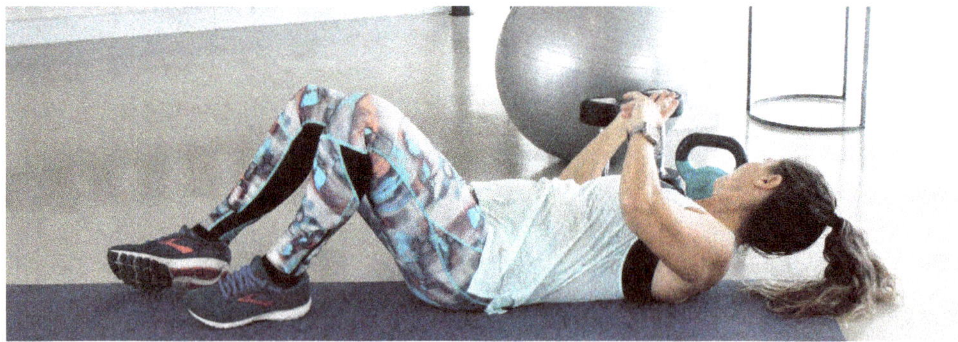

If you are going to try this guide independently, you need to consider these three points before you start out.

- Medical history (illnesses, injuries, medications, etc.)

- Athletic or fitness history (workout frequency, intensity, and duration)

- Goals (short and long term, recreational or professional, etc.)

Whether you are training for the first time, or are a seasoned athlete, or at the beginning of any training programme, anything more or harder than what you're currently doing will most likely stimulate progressive overload and adaptation. It is my aim through this guide to provide enough exercises for you to train with, using functional movement and targeting specific areas to develop so that you do not stand at the start line, or at your training session wondering how your legs are going to function without feeling like they are wearing two buckets of cement instead of shoes.

This guide is divided into **THREE PILLARS OF TRAINING** that are essential for building power as a menopausal woman:

- heavy lifting (and resistance training without weights)
- plyometrics
- sprint interval training

There are over 600 muscles in the human body and menopausal women have some specific considerations. The three main types of muscle include skeletal, smooth and cardiac, which provide the ability for us to breathe, get up, make coffee, drive to work, pick up the kettlebell off the floor (or the kids), stand and hold up a pointer at a presentation for hours on our feet, pump blood through our veins, and then still have energy to spend time doing the more enjoyable stuff like the movement or sports we love.

> BONES BECOME STRONG WHEN THE MUSCLES ATTACHED TO THEM BECOME STRONG

Bone changes are slow, much slower than strength changes. Research indicates that postmenopausal women who engage in a comprehensive training programme, benefit by maintaining a healthy body, bone density levels, and good mental health. Osteoporosis, the greatest ailment in older women, can be kept under control with exercise. Interestingly, The Department of Nursing, Physical Therapy and Medicine at the University of Almeria (Spain) did a study of exactly 5964 articles and research documents comparing randomized clinical trials that analysed the effects of strength exercises versus other types of interventions. All the results showed improvements in the strength of the legs and pelvic floor, physical activity, bone density, metabolic and hormonal changes, heart rate and blood pressure and a change in hot flashes.

I am concerned about menopausal females not doing strength training, because I know from personal experience that when we lose oestrogen as we age, we lose the anabolic stimulus of oestrogen and the ability to build muscle, as we did a decade before. It was so much easier in my early 40s!

With the menopausal journey, we lose neuro-muscular connection and fast explosive ability, so we really need to complement any of our high-intensity work, as well any plyometric work, with the ability to develop a very strong contraction, to maintain that muscle integrity which is our overall strength. You will do this by lifting heavy weights (scientific and reading references at the end of this magazine). NOTE: You will not bulk out!

BODIES

Earlier, I mentioned "metabolic syndrome" which is closely linked to overweight, or obesity and inactivity. If you have been diagnosed as insulin resistant, then this is also linked. According to the Mayo Clinic, "metabolic syndrome is a cluster of conditions that occur together, increasing your risk of heart disease, stroke and type 2 diabetes. These conditions include increased blood pressure, high blood sugar, excess body fat around the waist, and abnormal cholesterol or triglyceride levels." Please note that if you have one of these symptoms in isolation it does not mean you have metabolic syndrome, but it does mean that you are at risk for contracting one of the diseases. "Apple-shaped" bodies have abdominal visceral obesity and therefore carry a greater

risk of developing insulin resistance than individuals with "pear-shaped" bodies with subcutaneous fat accumulation. If you carry excess visceral adipose tissue this is often accompanied by fat infiltration of hepatocytes, a condition known as non-alcoholic fatty liver. Fatty liver can be reversed with simple lifestyle changes and a little training, do don't panic!

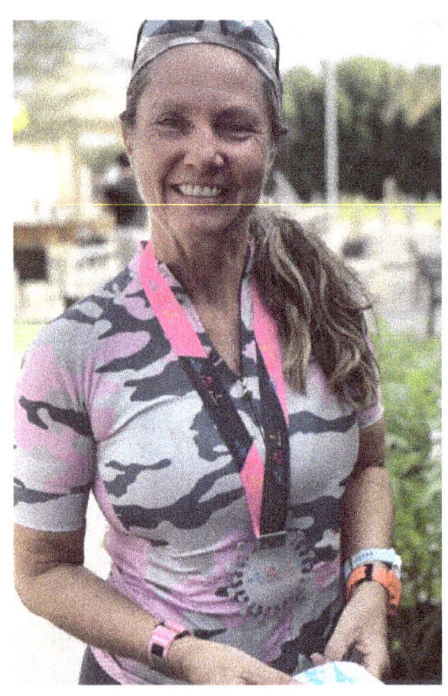

Now take a look at your body (as objectively as possible) and understand the risks you pose if you do not take action to make positive changes. Also remember that weight is just a number. You can be 70kgs of useful muscle (me, more or less) or 70kg of some muscle and "lard" (lard can be burned and that's why we are here!) While looking at your body, it's important to know also that there are 3 body types.

ENDOMORPH, ECTOMORPH, AND MESOMORPH, WHAT AM I?

If you are long-limbed, and not particularly muscular you are an Ectomorph (although you can still have "skinny fat").

WHY LIFT?

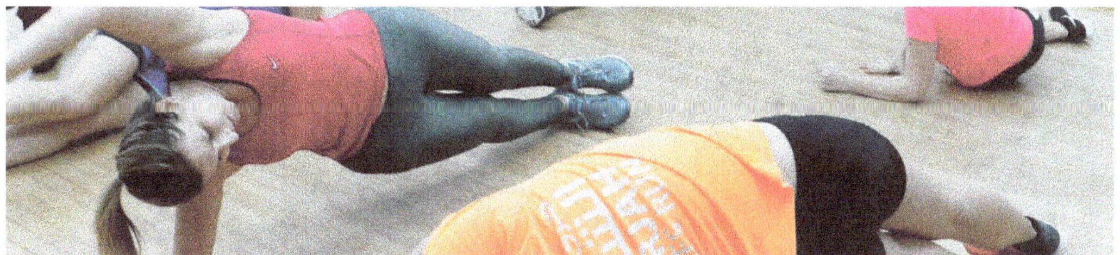

If you find it easy to build muscle and you are proportionally built, then you are a Mesomorph. If you are generally a bit rounder and store fat easily, you are an Endomorph.

If you're an Endomorph, here's the good news. CrossFit, high intensity work such as SIT/HIIT, weight training and moderate endurance training are great for you! This is a good reason to lift!

Strength training is the best way to generate muscle-making cells, and lifting heavy provides the strength-building stimulus you need as oestrogen declines. You also maximize your strength. The exercise routines in this guide should provide you with enough lift and resistance exercises to help you build and maintain strength, to be able to achieve optimal performance on race day, or for that specific goal you have.

The exercises can be performed at the gym or at home with minimal equipment and can be modified for all levels.

Importantly, the high-intensity sprint interval training workouts can provide the metabolic stimulus to trigger the performance-boosting body composition changes that our hormones helped us achieves in our premenopausal years.

GENERAL BENEFITS OF STRENGTH TRAINING

- Increased cross-sectional area of muscle (but not bulk)
- Increased power and strength production potential Increased metabolic rate and efficiency
- Increased joint strength and stability Increased bone mineral density Improved immunological status and cardiovascular health

STARTING TIPS

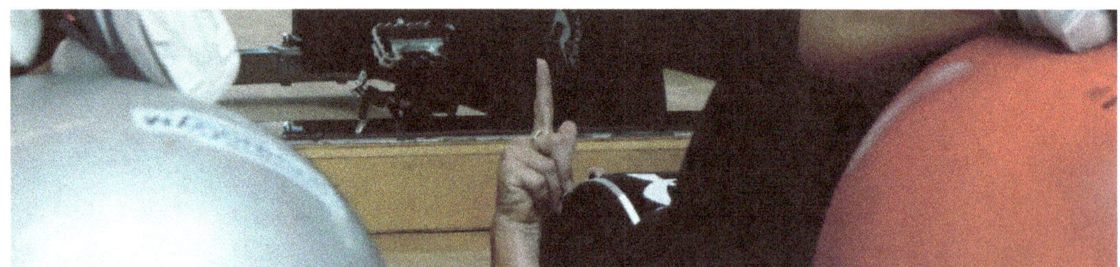

Included in this programme is a core routine, which can be performed as an alternative workout if you are short on time or as an additional workout during the week. This guide gives you many ideas to be able work out what's best for you in order to start your strength training regime. Not one size fits all, ever.

Safety is paramount. Lifting heavy is a sport with the potential to cause injury, so you need to be careful and make sure you get expert instruction on load and technique. Many gyms offer Olympic lifting technique sessions, I would recommend that you sign up to one of those if you can.

Learn each movement, practice without a weight first, start light, then increase your load.

Do not be afraid of the mirror! Check your posture regularly and write **BADASS** on the mirror in permanent market.

Train until you are fatigued, but not until you fail the lift. This will prevent injury (dropping weights on your feet or wrenching your back can ruin your season) Watch your range of motion and breathe through each repetition. Complete each movement to the full range of motion. If you cannot complete the move, go lighter again with the weight to maintain the quality of your movement.

If you have another training session scheduled on your strength day, then do the cardio specific discipline first (swim, bike or run or whatever). If you need to switch workouts around in your calendar, do not leave yourself too tired or sore to complete key sessions. For example, avoid a hard leg session before a speed run unless it is a specific HITT or plyometric session.

EQUIPMENT

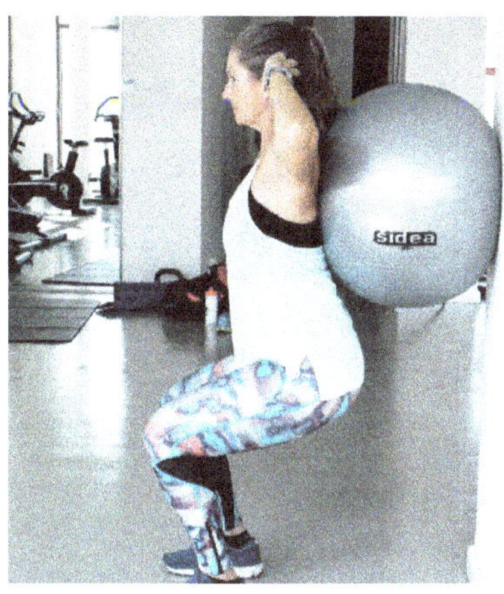 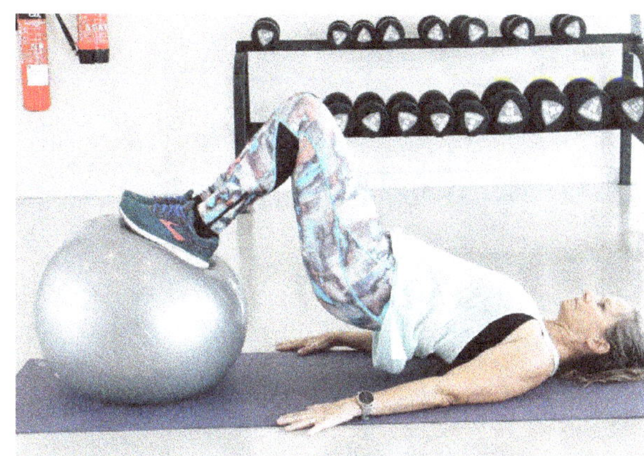

EXERCISE BALL

Make sure it is the right size for you. The following is a recommendation from Spine Health and is a general guideline for height correspondence to diameter of exercise ball is as follows (this is assuming average body weight is proportional to height).

If your body weight to height is larger than the average proportion, sitting on the exercise ball will compress it down more, so individuals usually should try using the next larger exercise ball size to maintain the 90-degree at the knee joint if you are sitting on the ball. If you don't have an exercise ball you can adapt your training to a bench.

Exercise ball diameter	Person's height
45 cm	5' and under
55 cm	5'1"– 5'8"
65 cm	5'9"– 6'2"
75 cm	6'3"– 6'7"
85 cm	6'8" and taller

DUMBBELLS

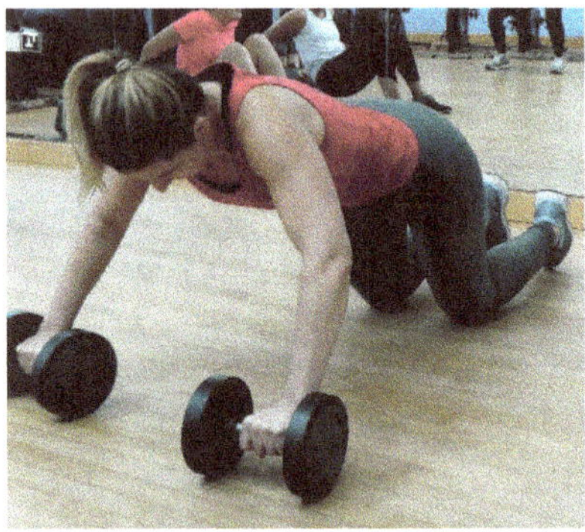 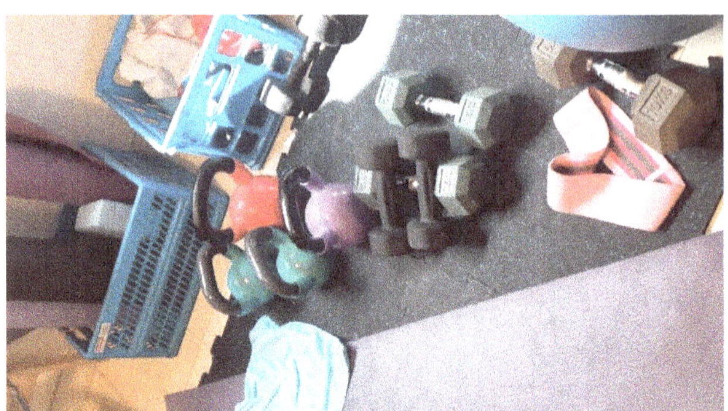

A range from 2,4,6, and 8 kgs should be enough to get you started.

At home I have the "hex" dumbbells as they don't roll and I can use them for press-ups. The rubber coating helps protect floors and other surfaces, and the contoured handle is easy to grip.

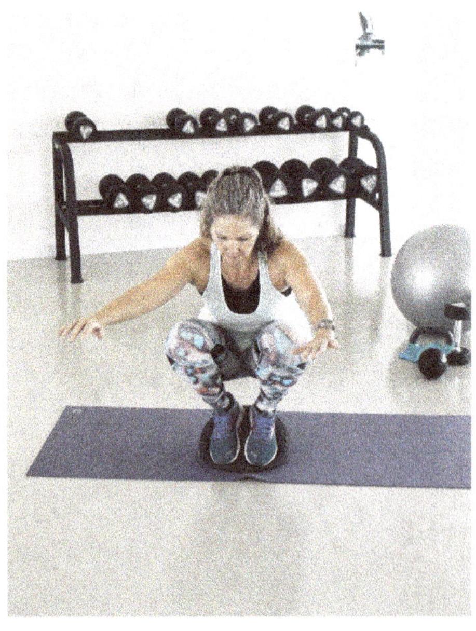

Plus, their hex shape makes it easier to stack them on top of each other for storage - my home gym is tiny!

Alternatively, if your dumbbells are the ones with discs at each end, you can use them for ab wheel roll-outs. The choice is yours.

STABILITY DISC

I use the PTP one (no affiliation), I just found it in my local sports shop. These force your body to stabilise your joints, like when squatting. I also sit on top of one at my desk!) There are 100s of exercises you can do with these, and when you buy it there is an instruction manual too.

Pump it up well....

KETTLEBELLS

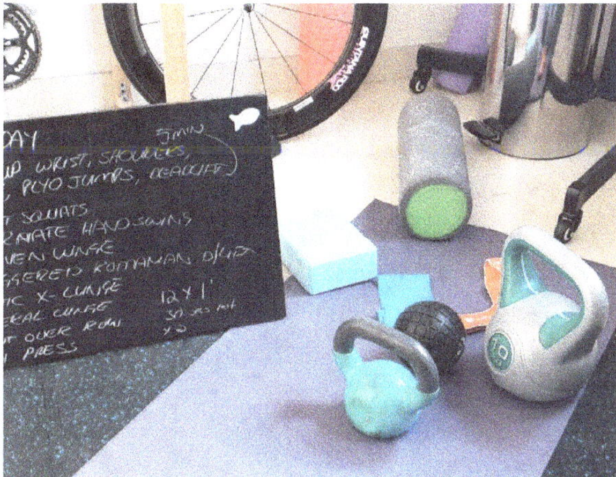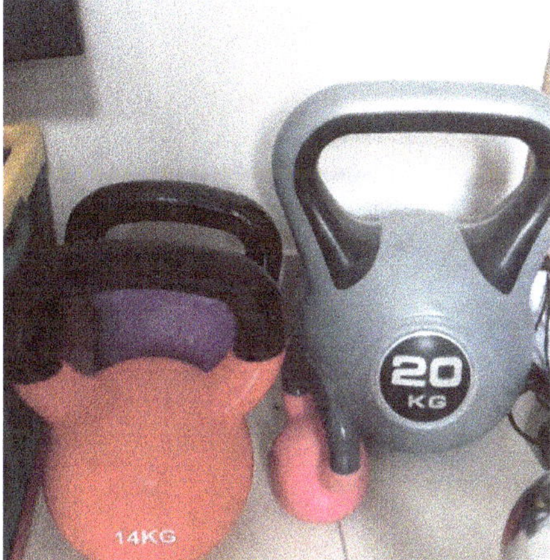

Kettlebells are my personal favourite. I use a minimum of a 4kg and up to a 16kg or 20kg depending on the exercise and where I am at in terms of my racing season. I am still working on going heavier.

Competition kettlebells are all the same size regardless of weight, which means they are ideal for practicing highly technical movements like the Turkish Get Up or high-repetition exercises. Cast iron kettlebells are often preferred by beginners because most beginners start with movements that require two hands on the handle – such as deadlifts, two arm swings, goblet squats – which can be difficult with competition kettlebells if you have big hands.

Note that this is not a weight prescription, you will need to taper it in. You might start with a 2kg kettlebell and work your way up to a 18kg kettlebell. It's important to know it is individual and it's about the intensity of your effort. As you get stronger, your lighter kettlebells will still be useful for mobility work, warm-ups and practising more advanced moves like the Turkish Get-Up. Lifting "heavy" is all relevant to your current fitness or strength point. What is heavy to me, could be light for others. If you are new to strength training, this guide will explain how to start, and some pointers as to how much to start with.

RESISTANCE BAND

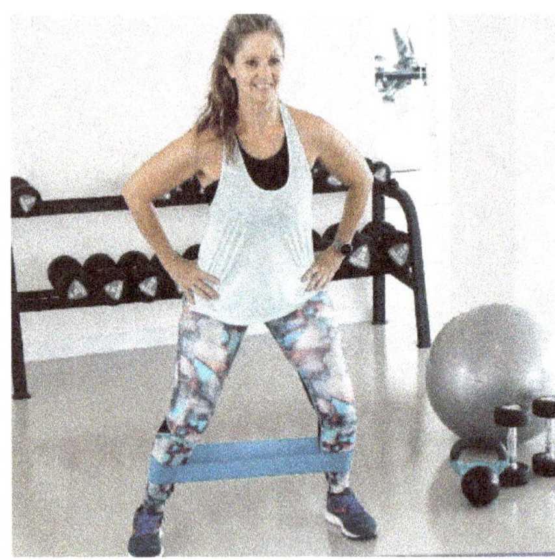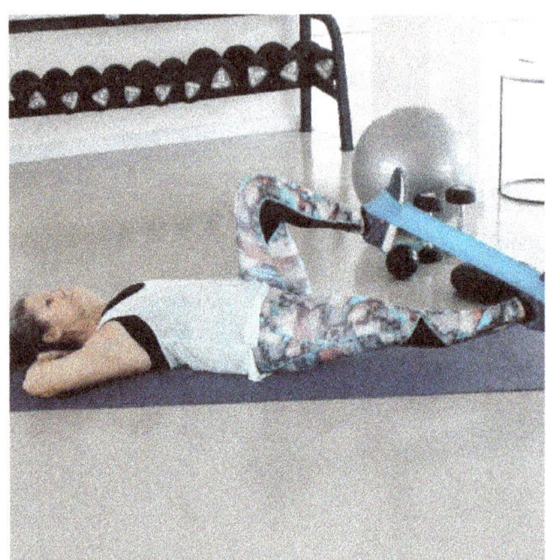

Check out bands which are adjustable so you can vary the resistance according to the exercise or those that come in a back of different strengths.

MAT

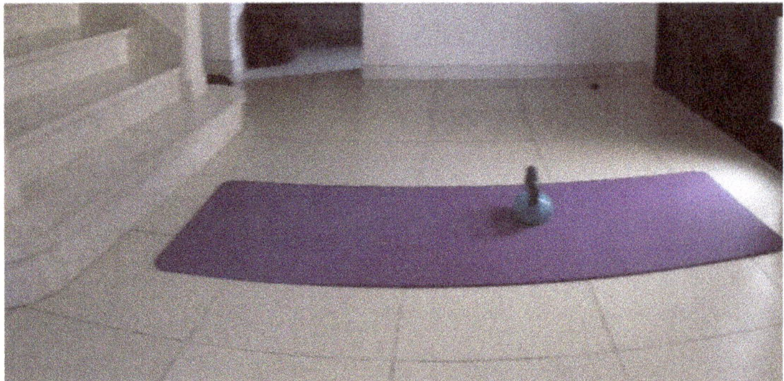

I always train on a mat as I train barefoot a lot. We tend to neglect our feet and focus so much on other areas that our feet that carry all the load are often not thought of. Ask me about plantar fasciitis, I had it for nearly four years!

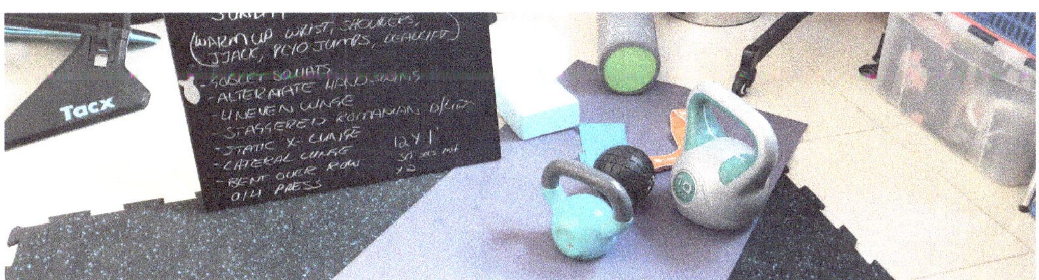

The explanations and photos you are seeing in this guide are all my own or of some my athletes (with their permission). There's no filtering, resizing or deletion of wrinkles, reduction of bloating etc.

What you see, is my body as it is now. I am a menopausal woman, and I am my age. Self-acceptance is a huge part of embarking on any fitness programme. Whatever your starting point is, or your mid-point, it's where you are. Be proud that you've invested in yourself to get to this point (contemplation, and perhaps ACTION). Be aware that there are so many fitness professionals online who are claiming to be "older" but are actually not, and also, there are many who are older and who are touching up their photos to iron out their imperfections.

Not here. So when you look at some of the moves, you will see some of my physical limitations, and perhaps a bit of flab here and there but who the heck cares. The point is that, like you, I am working on ME and everyone's journey is personal, and different!

Remember, warm up is crucial before you commence any strength training. You can mitigate joint pain and instability by performing a good warm up. This could be a jog around the block (or your corridor if you're in an apartment block), a row, some time on the bike, anything that is cardio related and gets the blood warm and the joints moving. If you do not have access to anywhere to run or a gym, you can do jogging on the spot, jumping jacks, inchworms, skater hops and all sorts. My "gym" at home is literally a 2.5 sqm space. You CAN make this work.

Let's get on to the exercises.

KETTLEBELL GUIDE

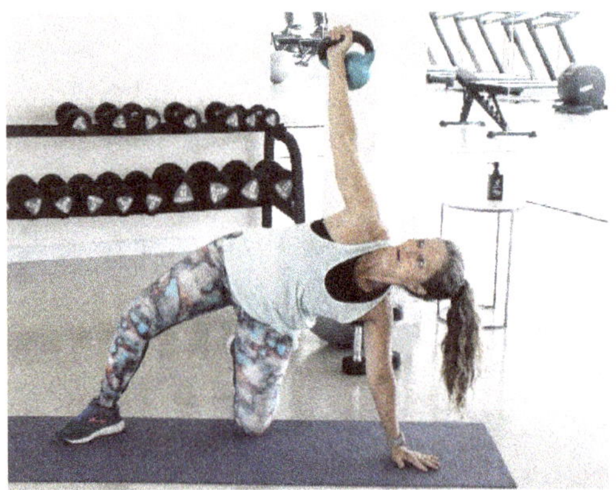

Kettlebells emphasize movements rather than isolating muscle groups. Therefore, they work many muscle groups at once, taxing the entire body. You can improve your strength and cardiovascular endurance simultaneously, and in as little as a 30-minute regular workout. There are also added benefits of enhanced stability, balance, coordination, and grip strength. The centre of mass of a Kettlebell is offset from the handle, making the Kettlebell unstable. This fluctuating resistance arm therefore forces the body to adapt in order to stabilize and control the weight. They are a highly effective conditioning tool, have been documented to burn up to 20 calories per minute. That would be equivalent to running a six- minute mile!

Many people have rehabilitated shoulder injuries and ailments through the combination of mobility, stability, and strength work using kettlebells. It is recommended that you check with a physiotherapist first before starting any kettlebell training.

In 2020 when there was a worldwide shortage of exercise equipment, some of us were using bottles of laundry liquid to "get sh*t done". If you do this, make sure it doesn't interfere with your swing. (More about swinging... shortly...)

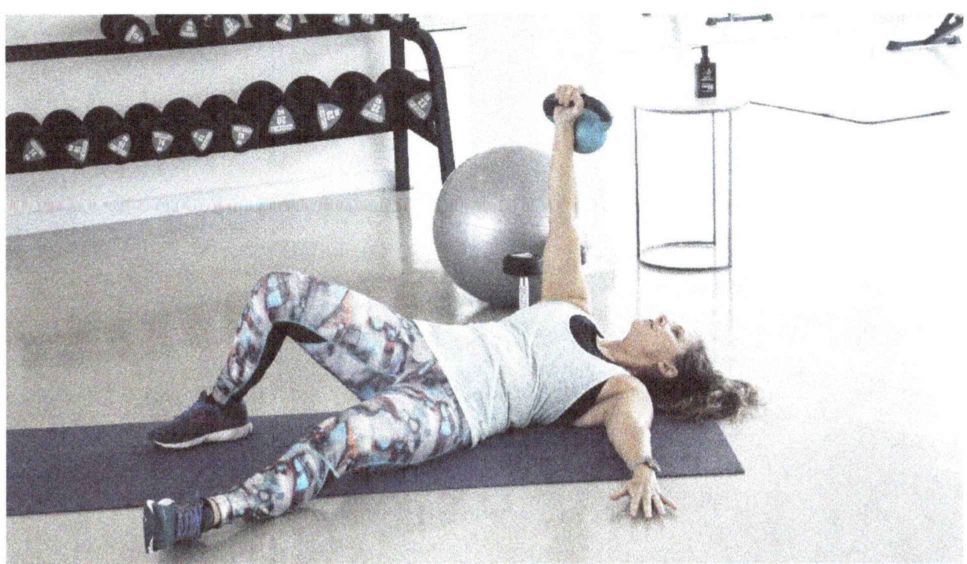

If you have a sedentary job, you might be suffering from poor posture. A simple 30-to-40-minute kettlebell workout 3 times a week will strengthen the posterior chain muscles (back, glutes, hamstrings) through proper technique and the gradual build-up of weight you are lifting.

Kettlebells are space efficient, making them perfect for home gyms and locations where there is no access to larger equipment such as barbells, machines, etc. They are definitely a fantastic tool for rebuilding strength and coming back to your regular training stronger than before.

In the information to follow, you will see a guide to some basic kettlebell moves. There are hundreds of different moves. Once you've mastered the basics then get online to Kettlebell Kings, KettlebellCentral, Greg Brookes (KettlebellWorkouts) and the inspirational Brittany van Schravendijk. I have done an online class using kettlebell flow, incorporating dance moves and music to suit. Create your own, get a friend, do it together!

REMEMBER: QUALITY OVER QUANTITY!

BASIC KETTLEBELL MOVES

- The Deadlift
- The Swing
- One Arm Swing
- Goblet Squat
- Split Squat Row
- Sumo Squat
- Two Arm Press (Overhead Press)
- Hang High Pull
- Turkish Get Up

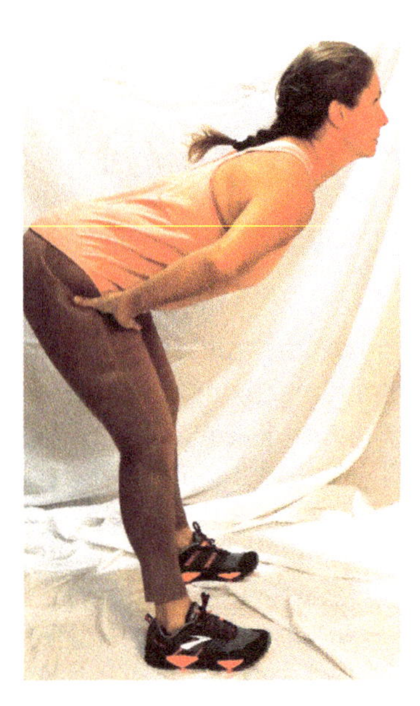

In order to use kettlebells safely and effectively, you need to learn the hip hinge movement first as it is the foundation of all kettlebell training.

A proper hinge involves primarily bending at the waist rather than squatting. The knees will still bend. Anatomy dictates form, therefore, everyone's hinge will look slightly different.

The length of the torso, arms and legs directly impact what the hip hinge will look like. A hip hinge looks like the move you would make when you close your car door using your butt, when you are holding all of your shopping or your sports bag.

Keep your arms and chest forward while you stick your hips out the back. Thumbs are placed together, tip to tip Hands are then dropped between the patella.

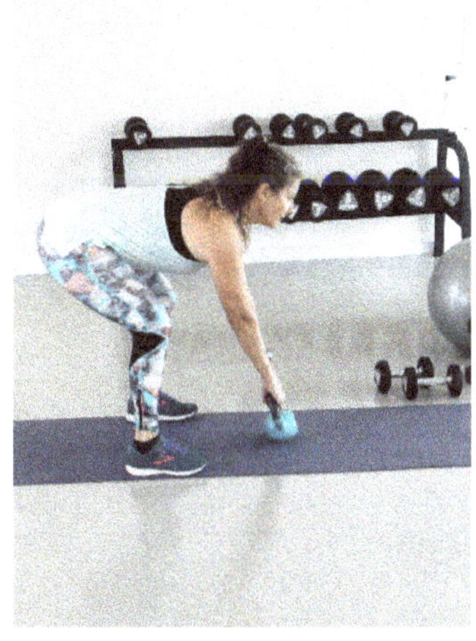 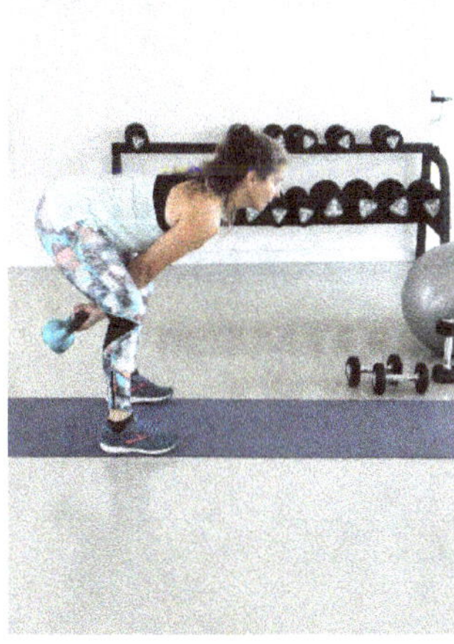 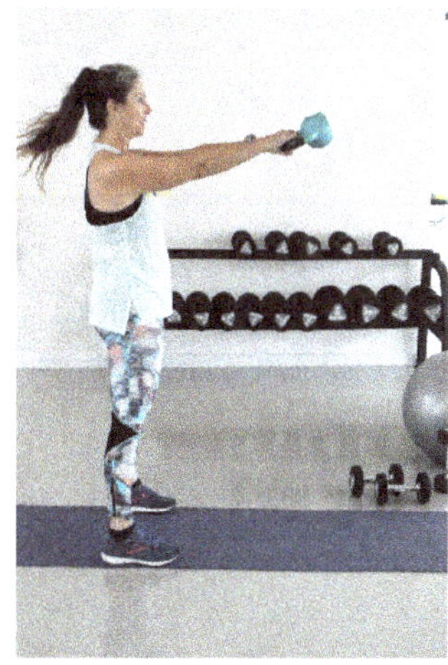

Establish stance using the thumbs method and place hand on thighs.

HINGE UNTIL THE TIP OF THE INDEX FINGER TOUCHES THE KNEECAP.

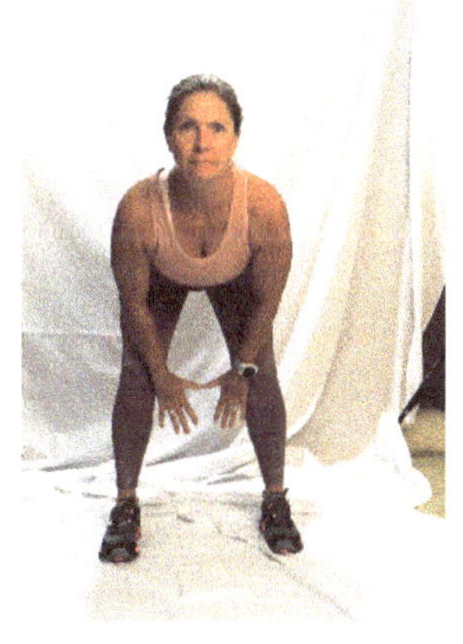

In this photo, the position is too low! Be sure to raise up higher.

This is the position the body should be in for most hingeing exercises. Remember, it is important to reinforce that the hips are moving horizontally rather than vertically. Vertical movement would be squatting. You keep your arms and chest forward while you stick your hips out the back.

Next, practice maintaining a neutral spine. This is perhaps the most important part of doing a hip hinge as it is the key to preventing injuries.

Adding a heavy load, and dynamic explosive movement to spinal flexion, is again putting yourself at risk for spinal injury. Remember, minimal knee bend, maximal hip flexion. Your complete movement should look like the above.

Several studies (including women!) show KB swings are a hip dominant exercise and the knee making the second largest contribution.

KETTLEBELL DEADLIFT

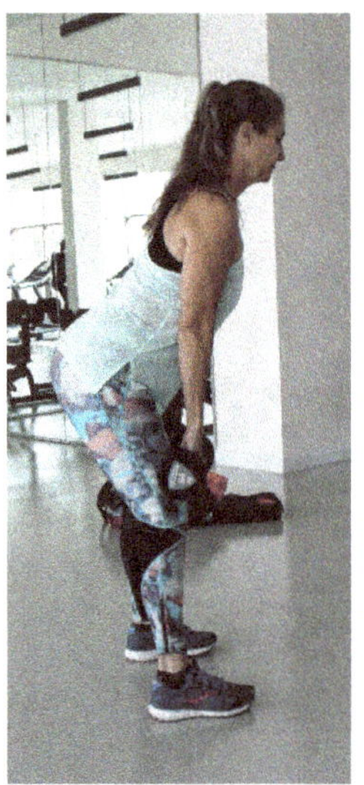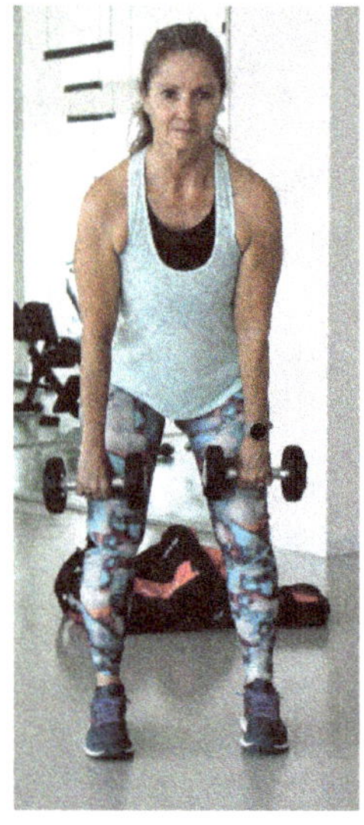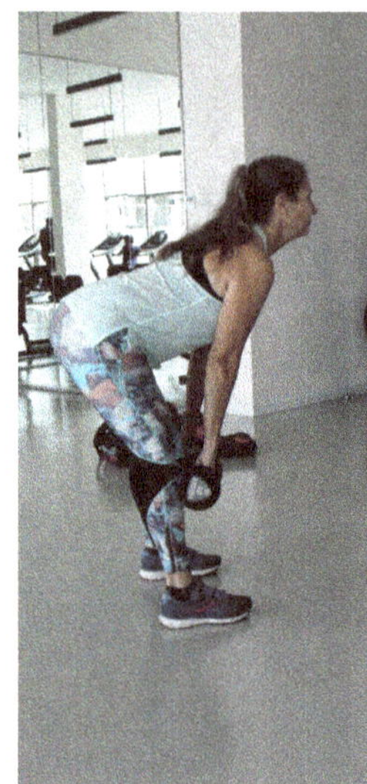

The deadlift is the basis for all bend patterns, whether it's picking something up off the floor or a kettlebell swing. Once you feel that you can perform the unloaded hinges, it is time to introduce the kettlebell (or dumbbell) to that movement. The deadlift is the basis for all bend patterns, whether it's picking something up off the floor or a kettlebell swing.

The most important element to remember for the deadlift is that the neck and spine should remain neutral, and you should push your butt back. The hips should remain at or BELOW shoulder level in the starting position. The back should not round, as this can drop the head lower than the hip and increase your risk for injury if you have not trained your back in this position.

Remember to drive through the heels and squeeze the glutes at the top of the lift to fully extend the hips. (When you squeeze your glutes, imagine that you're holding a Menthos in your butt cheeks. Seriously! And don't drop it...)

THE SWING

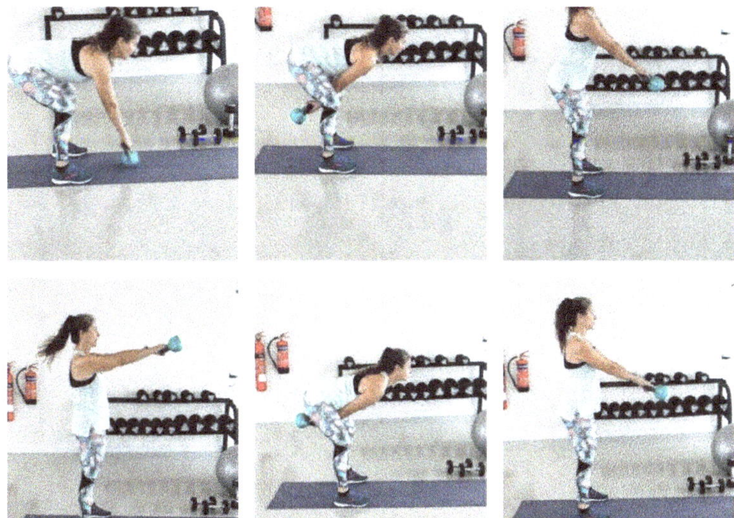

The Swing is an explosive kettlebell hinging movement, using the hip hinge that you have learned earlier. This movement trains powerful hip and knee extension and involves the muscles of your glutes, hamstrings, quads and lower back.

Also, it builds your grip! I find that I started to lose that with menopause and especially when I took a break from kettlebells when I was ill, I couldn't open a jar of peanut butter. That was the last straw....

Using the hinge movement previously learned, start off by doing the following steps:

- Stand over the kettlebell. The kettlebell should be directly under the hips and between the ankles.
- Slowly push the hips backwards, while maintaining vertical shins and a flat back
- Crush grip the kettlebell with both hands
- Engage the lats and upper back and take a deep breath into the belly
- Drive the hips forward and stand up while maintaining a neutral spine. Exhale!

SINGLE ARM SWING

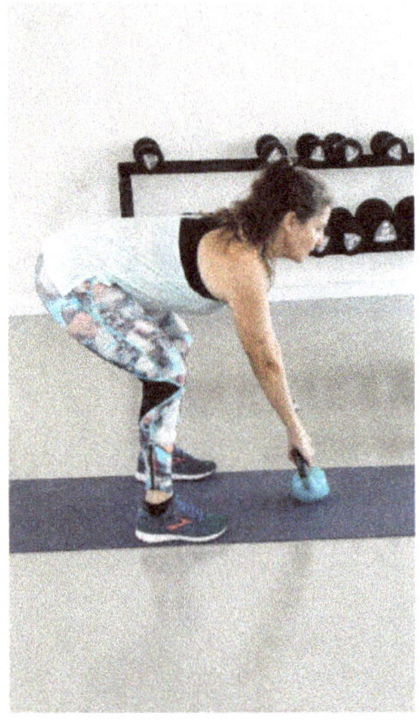 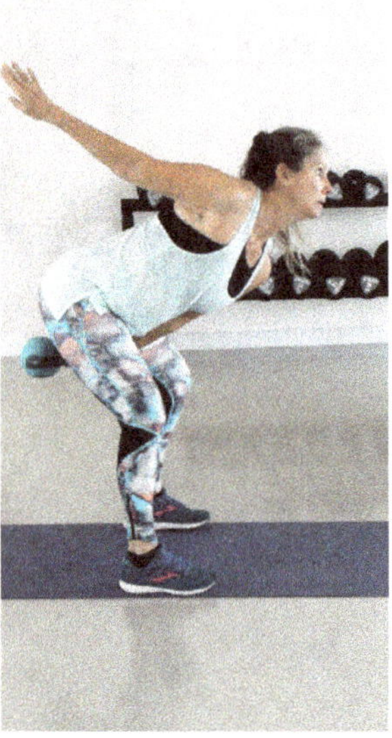 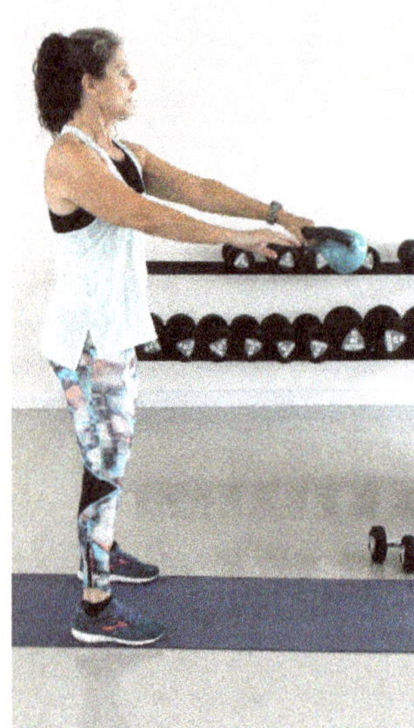

The single-arm kettlebell swing is a popular exercise emphasizing the muscles of the hamstrings, glutes, and back. Because you are only swinging with one arm at a time, it is also uniquely challenging to the grip and core muscles. It is often used to train explosive power, for aerobic or cardiovascular conditioning, or in SIT.

The movement pattern is nearly identical to the regular Swing; however, it requires more coordination and core activation to prevent rotation.

- Start with a kettlebell about 12 to 18 inches in front of you.
- Push your hips back, and squat slightly, as you reach forward for the kettlebell with one hand. Keep your shoulders higher than your hips.
- Grab the kettlebell and hike it back, pulling it high to your pelvis. Keep a neutral spine, your shoulders squared off, and your eyes on the horizon.
- Stand up tall and fast and swing the kettlebell to chest height. Exhale on top.
- Mimic the swing with your free hand to create power. Repeat.

GOBLET SQUAT

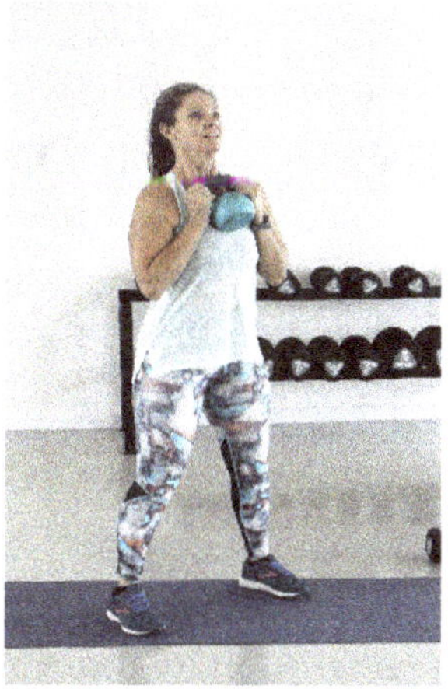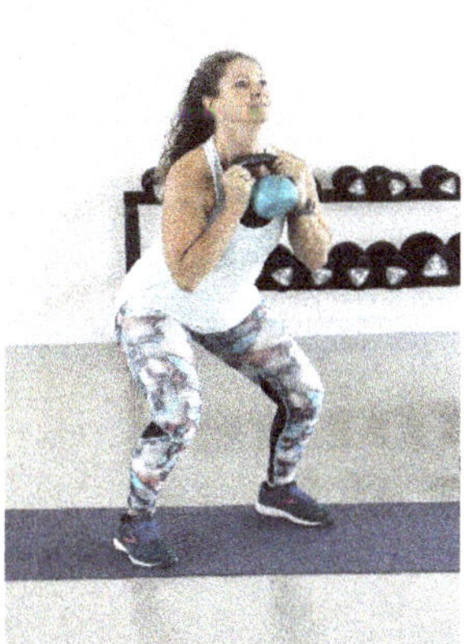

NOTE: You should hold air in the belly which will help to stabilize the spine during all the hinging and squatting movements. Many kettlebell sport competitors do the exact opposite as they exhale in the down phase. This helps to control the heart rate; however the kettlebell is being used as a fitness too.

Diaphragmatic breathing is safer overall for beginners and striving for the training effect from an increased heart rate.

The goblet squat is one the single best squatting exercises for general fitness. It builds strong legs and core. Adding a kettlebell in front of your body allows you to keep your torso more upright and puts you in an optimal squatting position.

If you find you can't squat without leaning forward, then try facing a wall and doing the squat. It will force you to keep your back upright. Keep your fingertips on the wall to support. By doing this you will learn to squat keeping your chest upright. If you squat leaning forwards, you can damage your spine.

To start, commence your squat with the kettlebell on the floor between your feet, grab with both hands and safely clean the kettlebell to chest level.

Hold the kettlebell by either side of the handle with your elbows close your body and the kettlebell touching your sternum.

Take a big breath and brace your core. Pull yourself down into a deep squat until elbows lightly touch the inside of your knees. Keep your chest up and weight toward the heels.

Drive hard through your heels and contract the glutes and reverse the movement while maintaining a neutral spine. Exhale about two thirds of the way up.

SPLIT-SQUAT ROW (SINGLE ARM ROW)

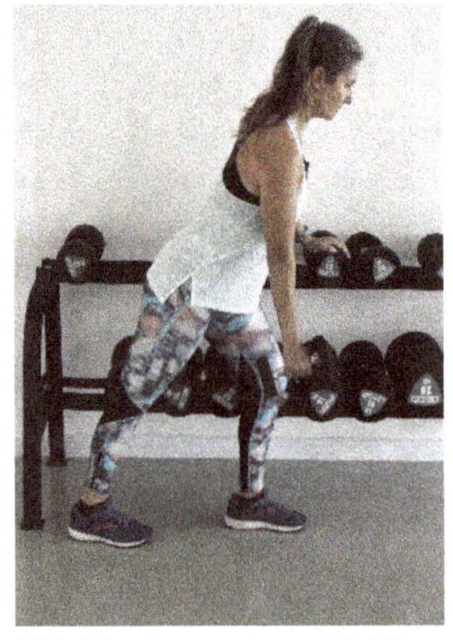 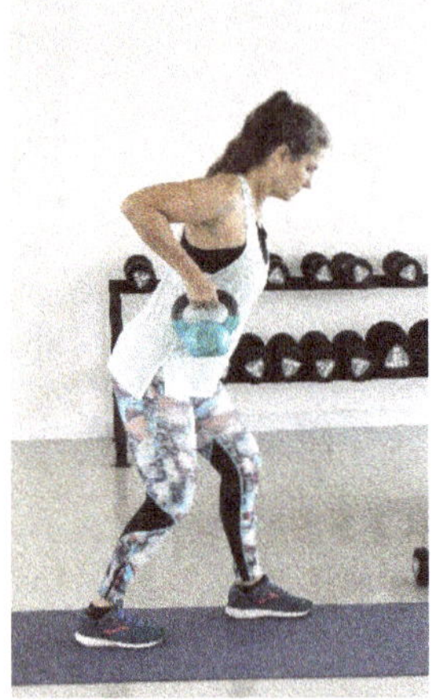

Start in a split squat position with the kettlebell on the side of the leg that is reaching back. Maintain a neutral spine with shoulders above or at the same level as the hips.

Grab the kettlebell handle, protract the shoulder blade to engage the upper back and lats, and then pull the elbow towards the belly button to lift the bell.

When the bell handle gets to stomach level, slowly lower back down to the starting position.

In these two photos you will notice that my hip is dropping to the right. I have lower back weakness due to poor core strength. I've been working on this over time. Make sure your hips are aligned and not drooping to one side when you do this movement.

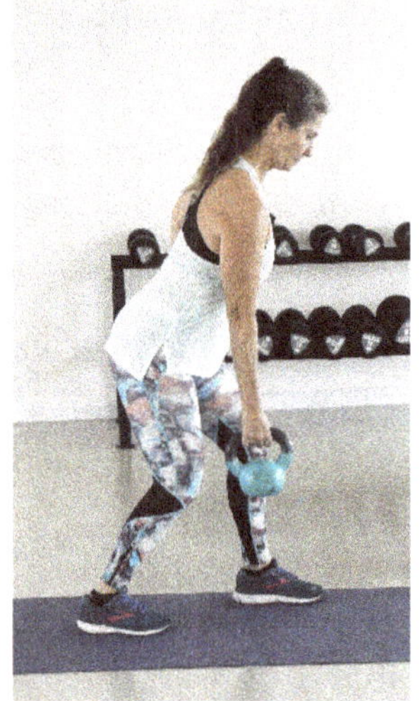

If you are just starting out with strength training, start with a 4kg kettlebell (or dumbbell) and work your way up.

Do not compromise your posture for heavier weight.

SUMO SQUAT

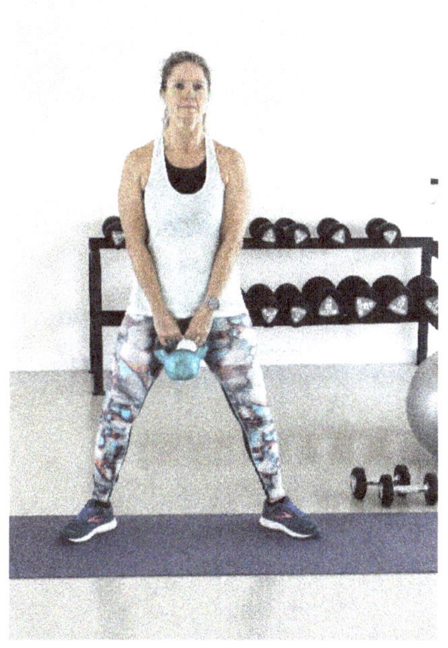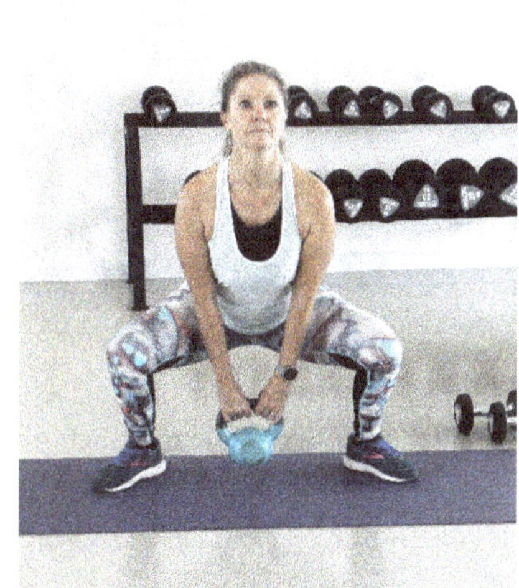

The kettlebell sumo squat is an excellent exercise primarily focused on the lower body with a particular flair for the quads. It is primarily performed by athletes in order to induce significant training stimuli in all the muscle groups of their legs, as well as to improve their explosive power, of which is a particular necessity in endurance sports. (Think of that sprint finish!)

Stand with feet slightly wider than hip-width apart, toes pointed out at 45 degrees, torso leaned slightly forward.

Hold the kettlebell in front of your pelvis with straight arms, and grip firmly.

Inhale as you bend your knees and sink your hips down until your thighs are parallel to the floor. Exhale and drive through your heels back to starting position.

Try to smile. I am not glum, really!

ONE OR TWO ARM PRESS (OVERHEAD PRESS)

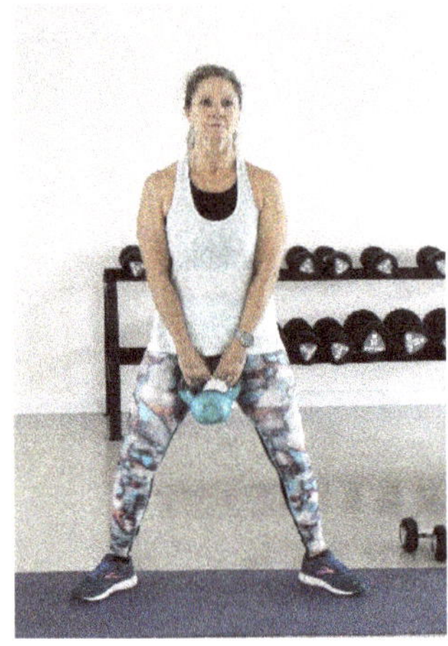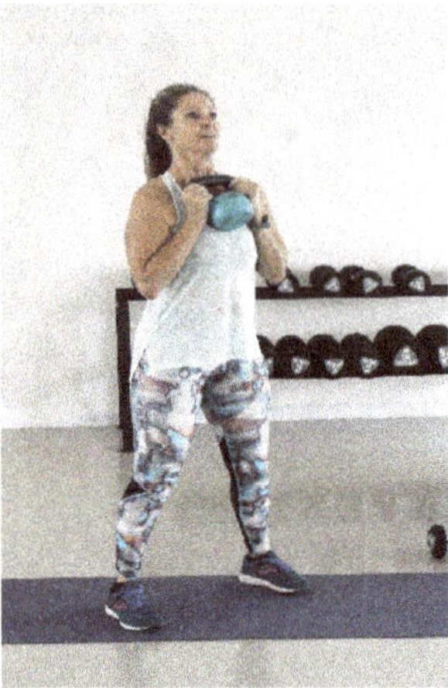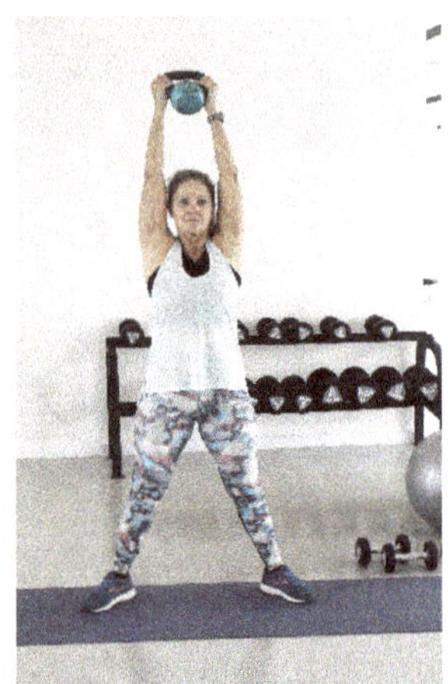

This exercise is great for increasing mobility in your upper back and shoulders. It can be used as a pre-pressing drill (warm up) or just to practice your pressing pattern. The kettlebell press is one of the staple kettlebell exercises. This movement develops your shoulders, triceps and to some extent your chest.

Follow these steps:

"Clean" (pick up and rack) the kettlebell. The handle should lay across the lifeline on your palm. Your thumb should be in front of your collar bone and elbow as close to your help as possible.

Squeeze the kettlebell handle hard. Tighten your glutes, and core.

Drive the kettlebell straight up. NOT out to the side, then up—remember the most efficient path when fighting against gravity is always in a straight line up and down… Lockout your elbow, unless you have an injury or condition that prevents this. Your bicep should be close to your ear. The kettlebell should be directly over your heels. Keep your core engaged and stay tight on the lockout.

Unlike the kettlebell press you are using your legs to perform more work. This can be more repetitions or involve a heavier weight. The kettlebell push develops your shoulders, triceps and to some extend your chest.

PUSH PRESS (OVERHEAD PRESS VARIATION)

Do as previous page but while leaving your hips extended and heels down, do a fast dip and explode up. DO NOT squat as this sends the weight of the kettlebell forward. Use your legs to lift the kettlebell. Drive the kettlebell straight up. not out to the side, then up—remember the most efficient path when fighting against gravity is always in a straight line up and down.

HANG HIGH PULL

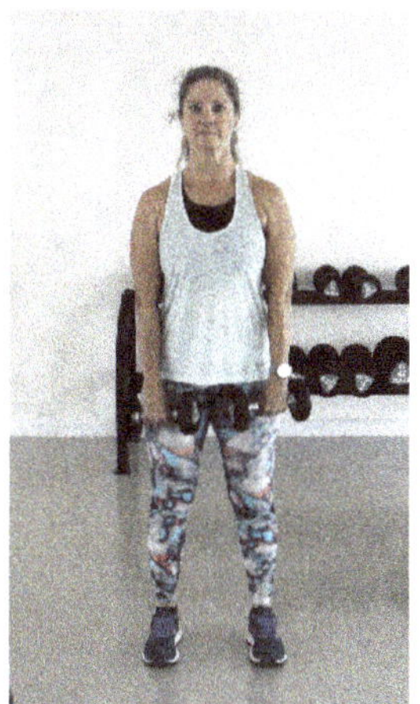
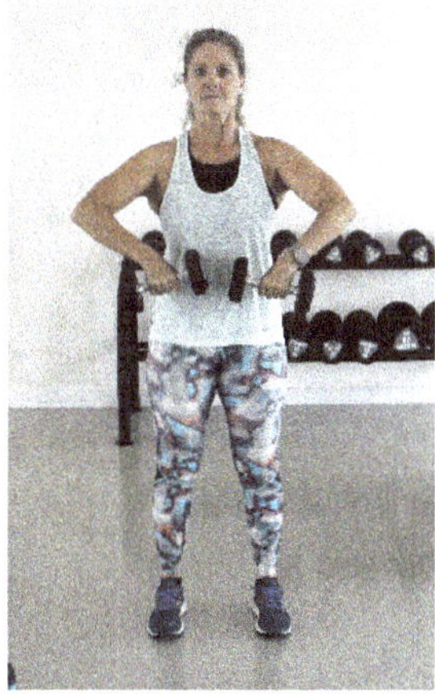
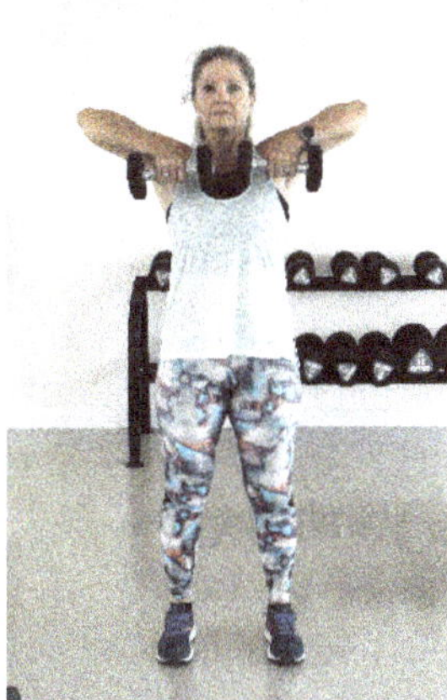

(Can also be done with dumbbells)

The kettlebell high pull exercise, like so many other kettlebell exercises, is a full body movement. Like the one-handed kettlebell swing the high pull works deep into the back of the body and so is excellent for improving posture and can be done with two arms or a single arm.

Start with the kettlebell on the floor between your feet. Your feet should be set slightly more than shoulder-width apart, at a 45deg angle to one another.

With your spine in a neutral position, bend your knees and lower into a squat position.

Using both hands, pick up the kettlebell and push through your heels. Engage your core as you move back up to your original standing position, pulling the kettlebell to hip level as you go. Raise the kettlebell until the handle reaches chin level, pointing your elbows up in the process. Lower the kettlebell back to your waist and get back into the squat stance.

THE WINDMILL

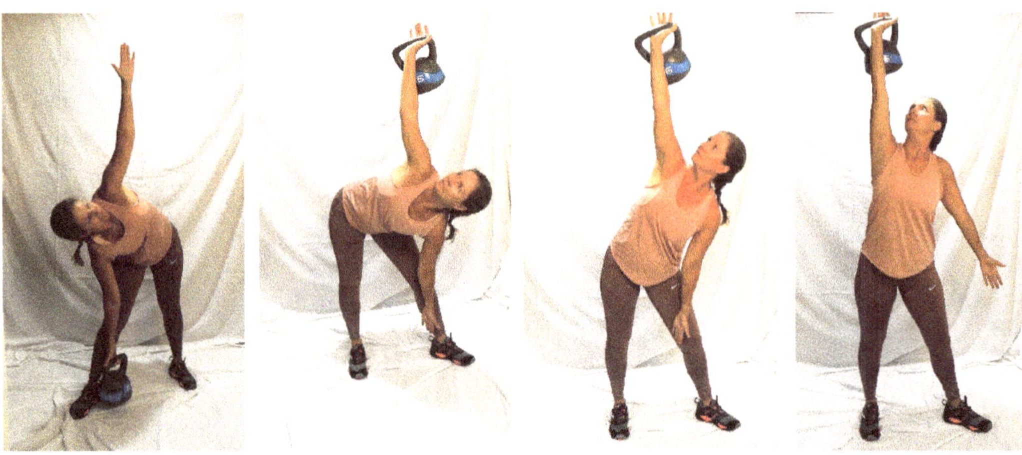

The kettlebell windmill is an excellent exercise for both stability and mobility. Gary Gray calls this term "Mostability". Some classify the movement as a core exercise; however, your spine only has a few degrees of lateral flexion, so most of the movement involves a hip hinge. The windmill will build hip mobility, hamstring flexibility, and shoulder stability. If you have a history of shoulder injuries or lack thoracic mobility this exercise may not be a great fit. It is also a good warm-up before doing the Turkish Get-Up, coming next!

- Stand with feet shoulder width. Take a small step forward and then turn your foot out. Do a "sassy" hip (push the hip back and to the side) and raise the opposite arm to the ceiling. Don't have your feet pointed in opposite directions.
- The other hand then goes down on the inside of your leg towards your knees. Touch the ground if you can! Do two or three times.
- Keep back knee locked and push backside towards the wall and your front knee slightly bent.
- Don't lunge forward, make sure hip moves backwards. (Use a PVC pipe if necessary get someone to hold it and keep contact with the pipe with your hip as you lunge).

Once you mastered this you can add load to the exercise, bottom, top, and both!

THE TURKISH GET-UP

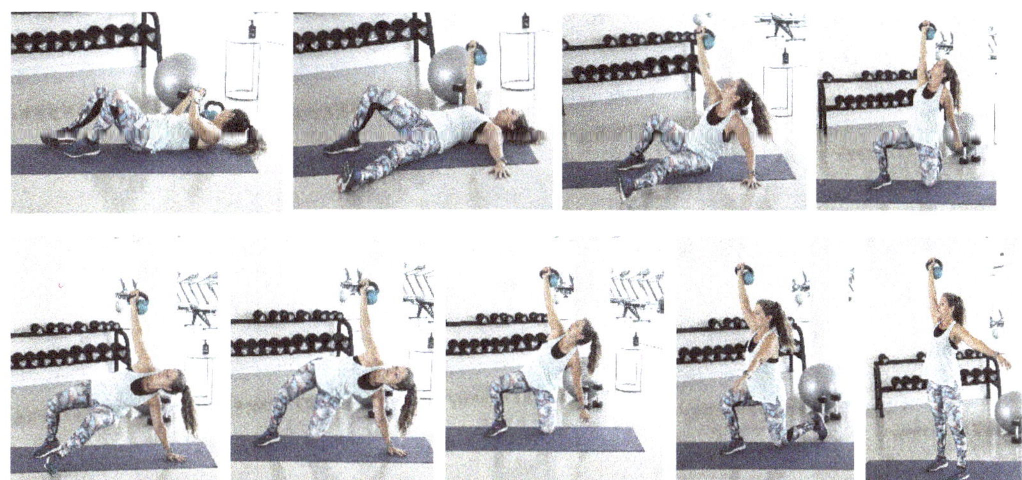

The Turkish Get Up is a full body exercise, with or without the kettlebell. There are many ways to perform the movement, and often coaches can make it overly complicated; however, it basically involves standing up with a load (after practice). The Turkish Get Up is best performed in a slow, controlled fashion. For best results take the time to own each step of the movement, rather than rushing through.

Here's a few of the benefits:

- builds strong, stable shoulders in multiple planes and positions improves core stability and strength
- improves hip mobility and trains hip extension
- develops basic and primal movement pattern, so it will help you move better! improves posture and it is a full body strength exercise.

For the first few times, practise just doing a "half get-up" until you feel strong enough to do the full movement.

See my YouTube Channel to watch a video. (@saraharriscoaching1476)

See next page for a full description.

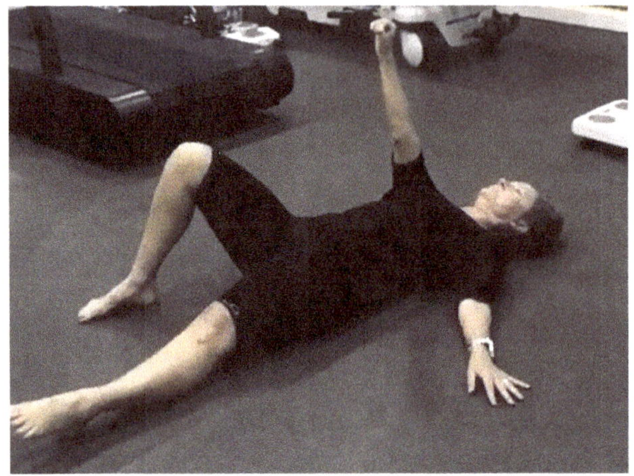

Grab your kettlebell safely and roll on your side. Start in a foetal position laid on the floor keeping your hands together by your chest. Your shoulder position is very important here and check when you are laid down that you raise your arm and pull your shoulder up and down (activating the shoulder).

Roll over and punch up the kettlebell, keeping one knee up, foot on the floor, (pull your heel into to your butt) and extend the other leg straight out on the floor. Drop your knee inwards and roll your hip, lockout your one hand with the kettlebell in the air) and roll to your elbow. Your other hand is now flat on the floor and you are resting on your elbow and forearm.

Raise up onto your hand from the elbow position, lifting your hips up off the ground like a bridge. Bend your knee and slide it through the body and now you are kneeling on it in the windmill position. Make sure wrist is straight and kb is across the palm. Keep your eye on the kb and lock out the arm.

Knee should be under your hips. Then straighten the body still holding the bell in the air with the arm locked out. With a windshield-wiper movement, straighten the back leg and stand up, feet together. Keep your eyes on the bell until you stand up and then look ahead. Now continuing the locked-out arm, go back to a lunge with your knee down, windshield wipe leg again at the back and go back to windmill position with your hand on the floor, locked out arms, hips raised and slide your leg back through and sit. Keep your eye on the kettlebell. Lower yourself back down.

Repeat. Try 5 each side to start…

RESISTANCE/STRENGTH TRAINING

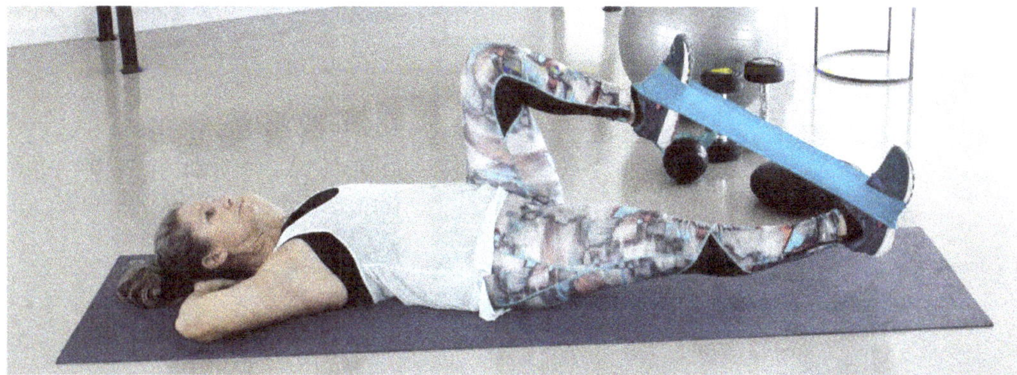

Just like during SIT (High-intensity Sprint Interval training sessions) and Plyometrics, you need to be working hard and not just using light weights 20 times. Women in menopause have a serious decline in sex hormones and lean muscle mass due to their ageing bodies. This type of exercise will build muscular endurance (seen often as ME in training programmes) however at this juncture of your life you need muscle strength. If you are starting out with strength training, then ME training will be needed for 4-6 weeks for preparation then switch to heavy lifting.

Heavy lifting means a few repetitions of times (like 3-6), including your body weight. If you do the traditional 3 sets of 10-12 repetitions you will create tiny tears in your muscle fibres which then repair, making your muscles bigger (hypertrophic). This can increase the amount of lean muscle you have BUT it will not stimulate satellite cells and replace the muscle and strength building stimulus that you are losing as your oestrogen declines.

Another reason why you should be heavy-lifting is that it will increase your metabolic rate, which means you will increase the number of calories you're using at rest (yay!). It also improves your posture and stability, which are specifically becoming an issue at the onset of menopause.

Your PT should only be giving you the traditional 3x10 (or 12) reps of lighter weight if you are starting out and building muscular endurance first.

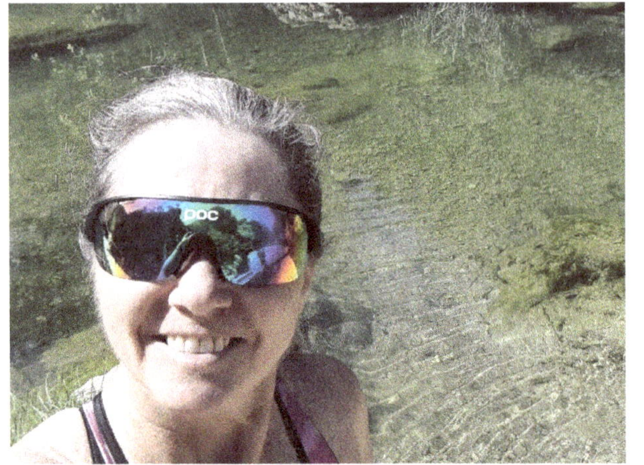

I personally suffer from joint pain particularly in the lower back, and instability. My chiropractor is always reminding me to do more core exercises and stability work. "Work from the ground upwards", he says. How can you expect to put your body through 100s of miles on the bike without working on the basics first?? (yeah, I know).

During perimenopause it is possible that you will have higher levels of inflammation and you lose a bit of the strength and tension in your tendons. I had plantar fasciitis for years! (I may have already mentioned that – meno-brain is not covered here). My physio said the same thing as Dr Stacy Sims - LOAD IT. Stimulate your tendons by loading with weight to increase their tension, which in turn will improve your overall stability and increase muscle strength to support your joints. Water running can help a lot with feet or leg injuries.

Heavy lifting also builds stronger bones and improves bone mineral density. You can get a DEXA scan to see how dense (or strong) your bones are. Start your lifting programme and check again after six to twelve months. See any difference?

If you have high blood pressure, heavy lifting is the way forward. It improves your cardiovascular health by increasing your vascular compliance giving you improved blood pressure control, and bloody flow to and from your muscles and skin.

Lifting heavy weights will improve your body composition. I am not saying that I ended up with the perfect body and I am very much always a work in progress, however the reduction of body fat is visible, and I cannot begin to explain the positive emotional gains as well.

Being stronger, helped me to run and bike faster, it helped my libido, it gave me more confidence to stand by the pool, because there's no beautiful body like a strong and confident one. With scars. And cellulite. I love what my body can do for ME.

WARM-UP AND LOWER BODY

ROLLING

Let's get started with some lower body exercises. Lifting heaving will not happen overnight and can take a few months to build up so please begin carefully. If you are new to strength training, start with two or three sets of only 10 to 15 repetitions. This will build the muscular endurance that I spoke of earlier. Give it about four to six weeks, and then decrease the repetitions and start increasing the weight and go to 6-8 reps. Remember, if you are lifting a kettlebell of 4kgs and then go to 8kgs, that is double the weight! Be cautious about how much you increase by. If your posture is compromised, go lower. Consistency in this process, is key. If you skip your sessions for two weeks (for example), that does not count towards your four-week period!

Start ALL workouts with a warm-up and mobility. Roll out your muscles and do "90/90" hip openers. For 90/90 flow moves, check out MEAUXTION on YouTube. Yes, he is a bloke. BUT, his 90/90 routine is brilliant and I use it on my athletes.

There is a realm of information available online and not all of it can be included in this book. So to start with, here are some rolling and band work ideas. On my YouTube Channel there is a short video to follow. If you flex your knee joint while rolling out your quad, it will dig in (floss) deeper! OUCH.

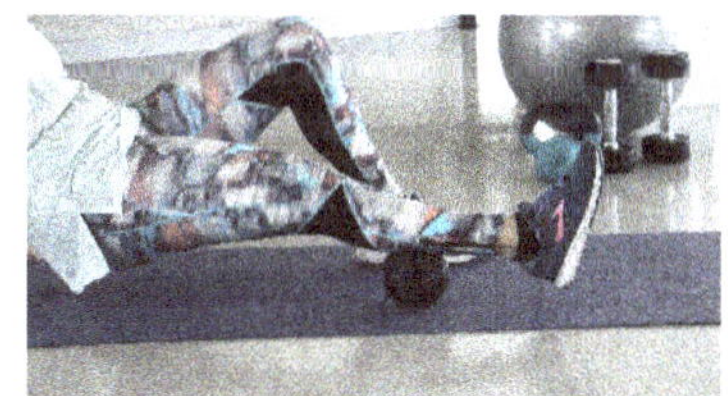
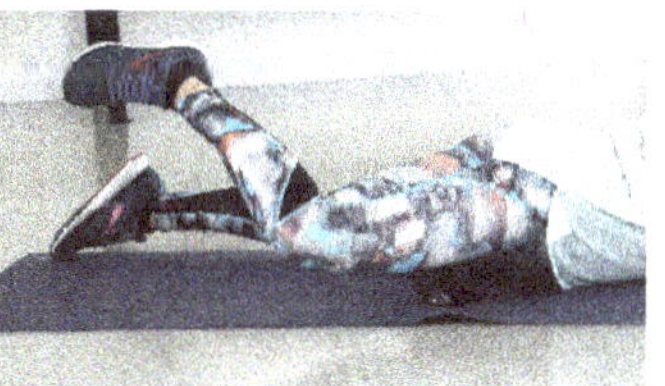
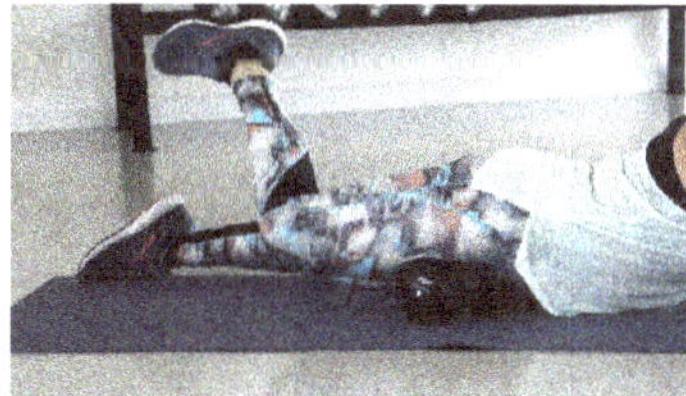
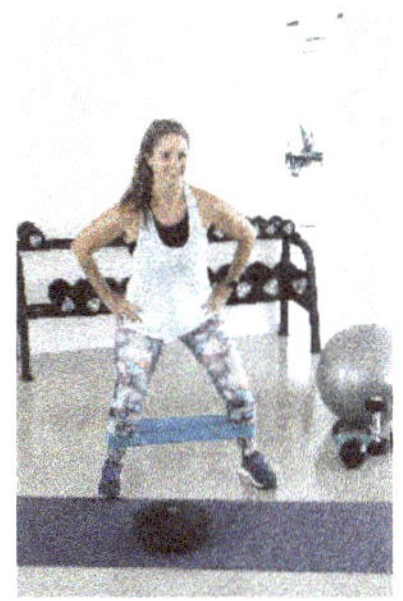
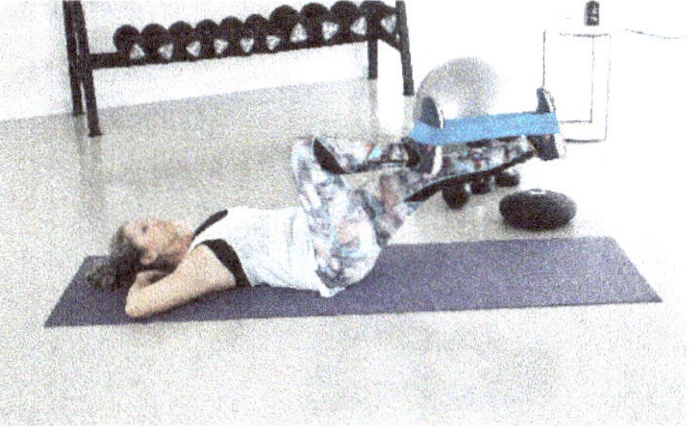

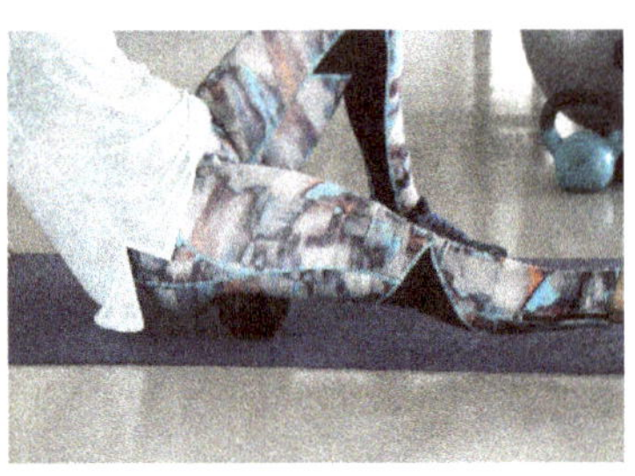

BALLS

Roll and floss all your joints with a ball. Where it hurts, pause!! Get in there. Do this before exercise and afterwards. Tissue care is key to future mobility and muscle repair.

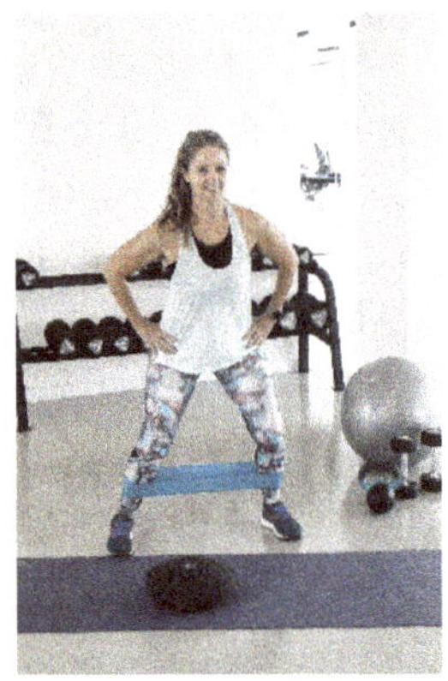

BAND WALK

In a 45-degree squat position, walk sideways, keeping the band taut.

BICYCLE BANDS

This exercise helps with strengthening of your hip flexors. "Bicycle" with the band across your feet, making sure you fully extend the leg each time. Keep your head on the floor.

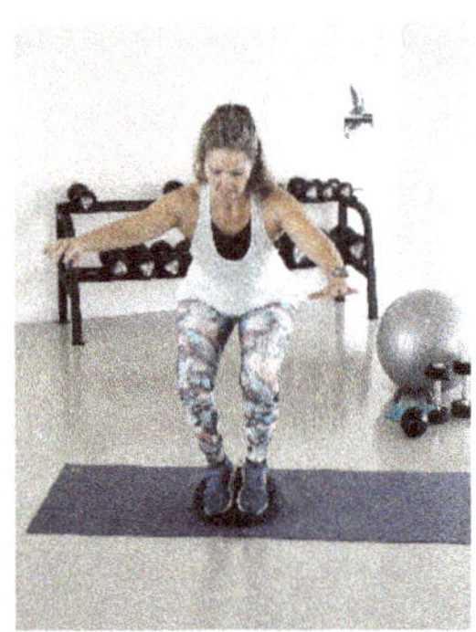

BALANCE

Get a stability disc and warm up your joints by squatting on a stability disc.

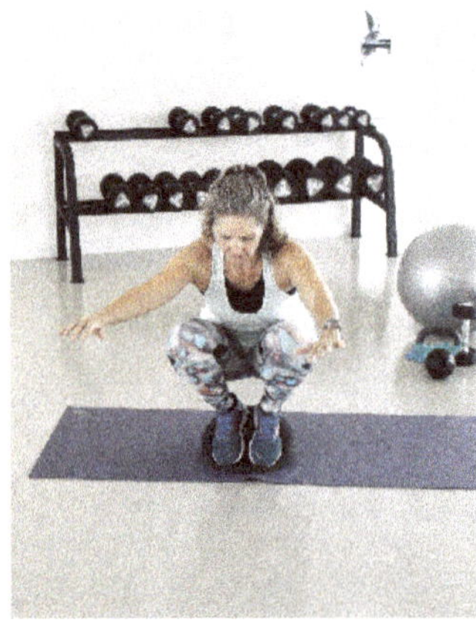

EXERCISES – LOWER BODY

- Isometric Wall Squat
- Soleus Wall Squat
- Stability ball crunch
- Bulgarian Split Squat
- Split Squat
- Weighted Calf Raise
- Weighted Calf Raise with a Dead Lift
- Back Extension with exercise ball
- Reverse Back Extensions
- Double Leg Raise
- Horizontal Bicycle

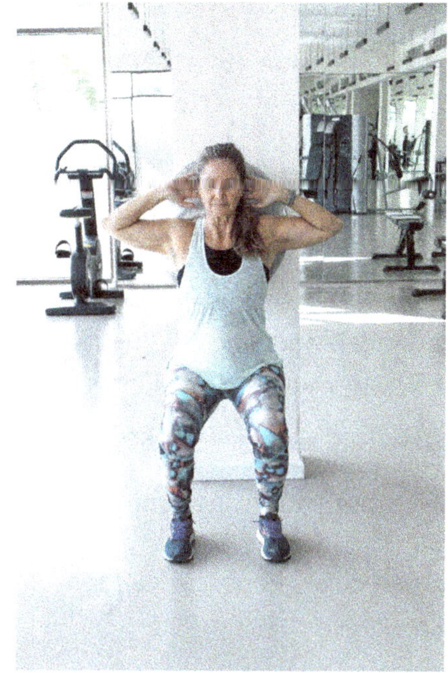

These exercises are mainly posterior chain, with a bit of abs mixed in. You will need your exercise ball, some dumbbells or kettlebells, and a mat. Make sure your exercise ball is well pumped, as the one that was in our gym on the day of photography was clearly not!

ISOMETRIC WALL SQUAT

Stand and squeeze the exercise ball between your lower back and a wall. Lower into a squat (as if you're sitting into a chair), letting the ball roll up your back until your knees are bent 90 degrees. Your knees should not be forwards of your toes. Push down into your heels and hold for 5 seconds and return to your start position.

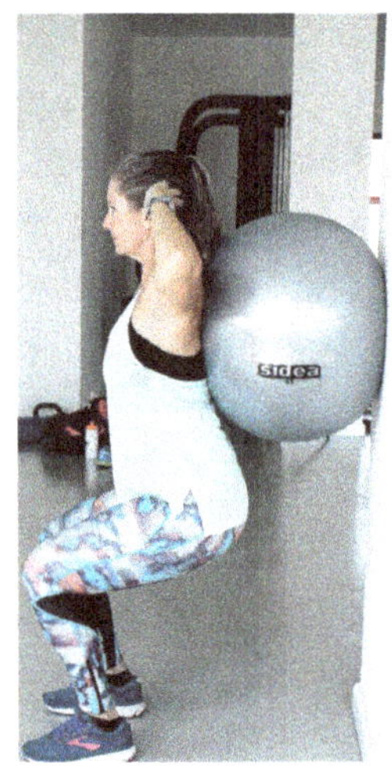

ISOMETRIC SOLEUS WALL SQUAT

This is not your typical wall squat but is effective for working the soleus muscle in particular if you are suffering from plantar fasciitis.

Stand against the wall and lower yourself to about 45 degrees, then raise up on to the balls of your feet and hold for 10 seconds, and slowly come down. Repeat.

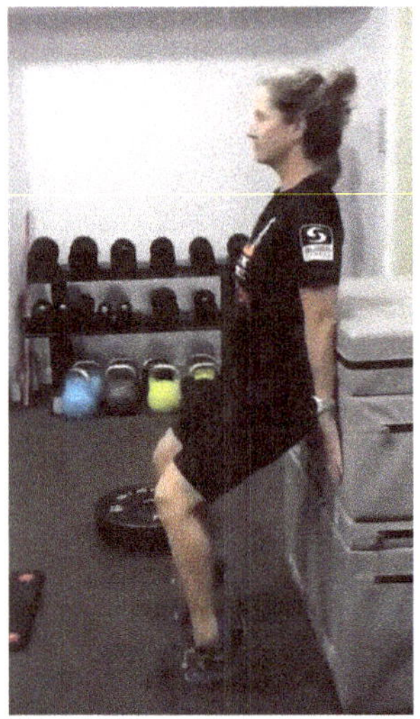

STABILITY BALL CRUNCH

Lie faceup on the ball, with the ball under your low back. Keep your feet on the floor, hip-width apart, and fingertips behind your ears.

Brace your core, tighten glutes, and slowly crunch upper body upward, raising shoulders off the ball and tucking your chin to chest. Slowly

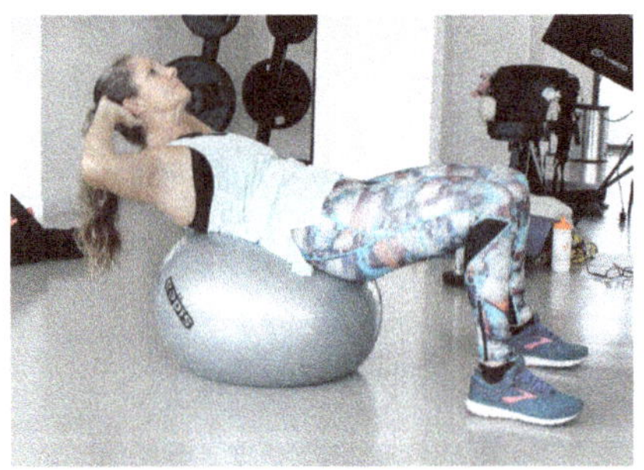

 lower upper body down to return to start.

BULGARIAN SPLIT SQUAT

You can do this exercise with your foot balanced on the exercise ball (harder), or on a bench.

The aim is to try and drop your knee at the back, while performing a single leg squat position at the front. The knee should not go over the toes.

Try without weights first, then add the dumbbells.

You'll place one of your feet on a bench behind you, but you may need to hop your front foot around a little bit to help you find the exact position that feels best.

SPLIT SQUAT

My running coach has said time and time again not to overreach when doing a split squat, and indeed, when running!

Split squats have many explanations over the internet; however, my tried and tested position is as if I were starting a running gait or movement.

Start with your feet together and lift the knee upwards. Lean forwards and land on your front foot. From this position, do your squat, then push back

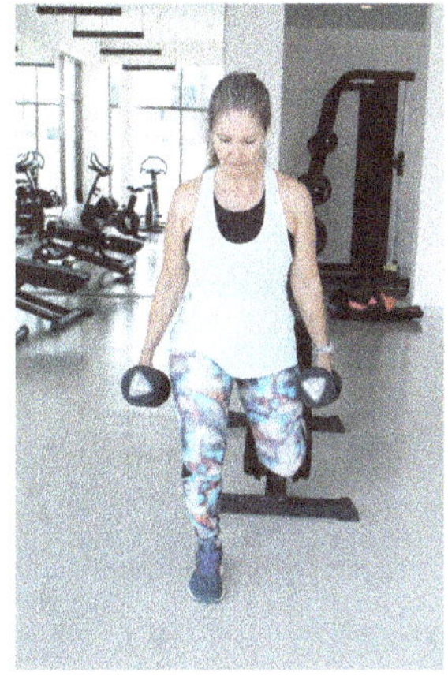

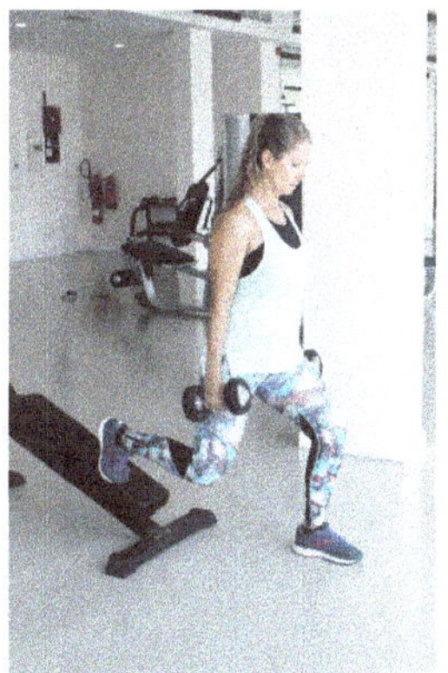

up into the starting position. The more stability and mobility you have, the deeper you will be able to squat

Make sure the front leg does not bend more than 90 degrees. Your back leg should be aligned with your hips, and not behind your foot in the front.

CALF RAISE WITH AN OPTIONAL DUMBBELL

Stand straight and engage the core.

Raise up slowly on to the balls of your feet, and slowly down. If you find this difficult using a dumbbell, do it with no weights at first and build up to carrying weights.

WEIGHTED CALF RAISE (WITH A DEADLIFT)

The most important element to remember for the deadlift is that the neck and spine should remain neutral, and you should push your butt back. The hips should remain at or below shoulder level in the starting position.

The back should not round, as this can drop the head lower than the hip and increase your risk for injury if you have not trained your back in this position. Remember to drive through the heels and squeeze the glutes at the top of the lift to fully extend the hips.

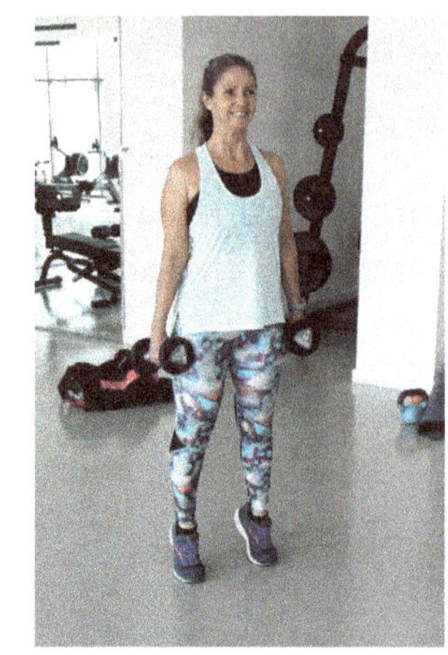

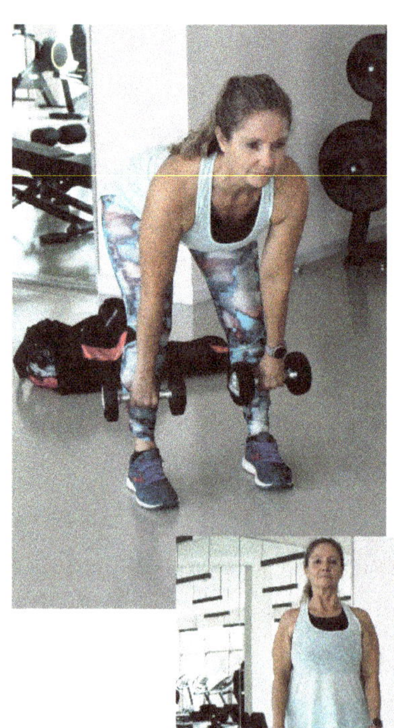

Deadlift, and raise up slowly on to the balls of your feet, and slowly down Then hip hinge and lower the bells to your mid- shin and stand up again.

BACK EXTENSION WITH EXERCISE BALL

Roll out with the ball until your hips are on top and anchor your feet to the floor. Engage the glutes and lower back and raise upwards, with your hands behind your head. You might only be able to do a small raise to start with, and this will get easier (as you get stronger). Lower the body again to the starting position. (Yes, I did cheat and had my foot against the wall I discovered my trainers did not grip this gym floor.)

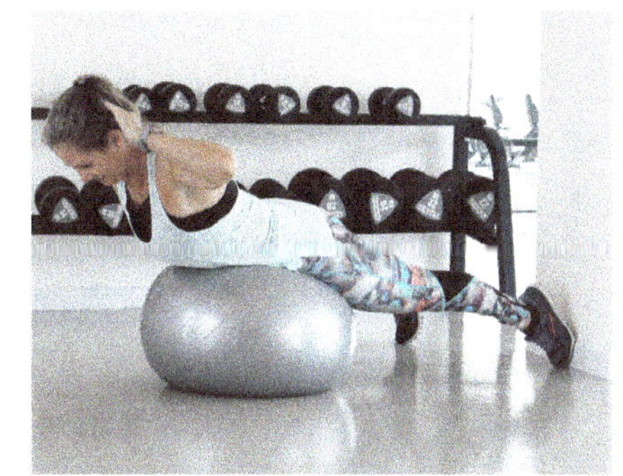

REVERSE BACK EXTENSIONS

I love these. Prop yourself up on your elbows with the ball under your pelvis. Engage the core, keep the feet together and legs straight (but soft). Lift upwards slowly enough to feel the back engage, and lower down. Repeat.

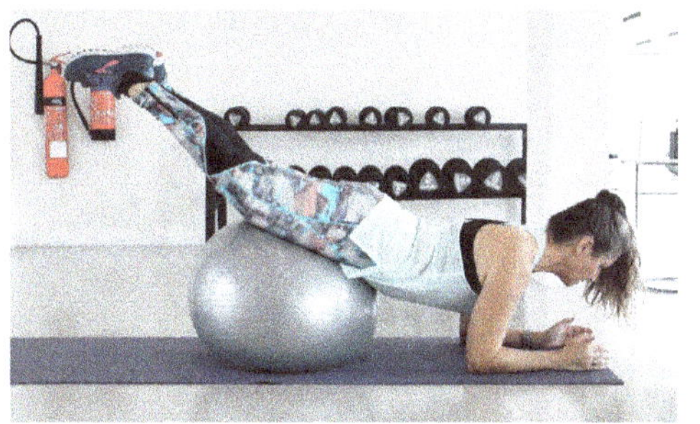

DOUBLE LEG WINDOW WIPER

Lie flat on the mat, press your lower back into the floor. Raise your legs, keep your feet together and drop your legs right to left. keep your shoulder blades on the floor and control the movement. Don't let your feet touch the floor.

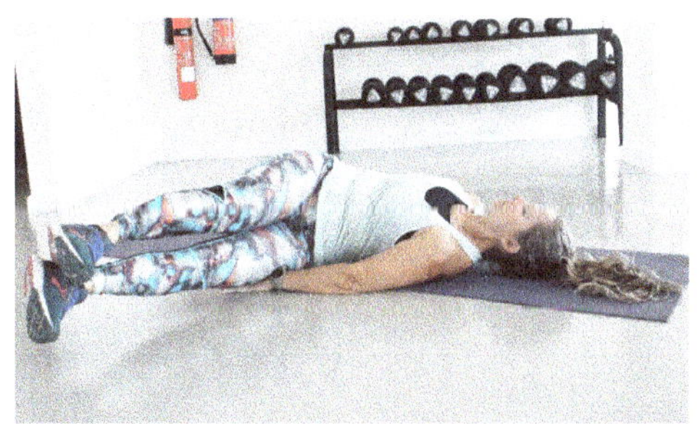

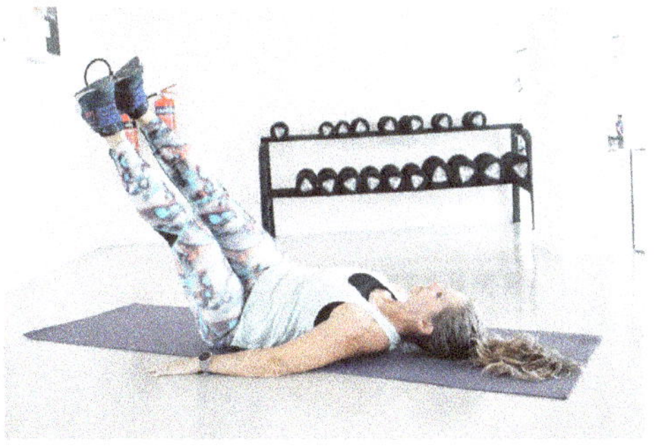

HORIZONTAL BICYCLE

With this exercise, you can work the obliques too by aiming to touch your knee with the opposite elbow. Remember to squeeze your lower back to the floor, engage the core and extend your "pedalling leg" completely outwards, and return.

Try to get your shoulder blades off the floor when you do this exercise.

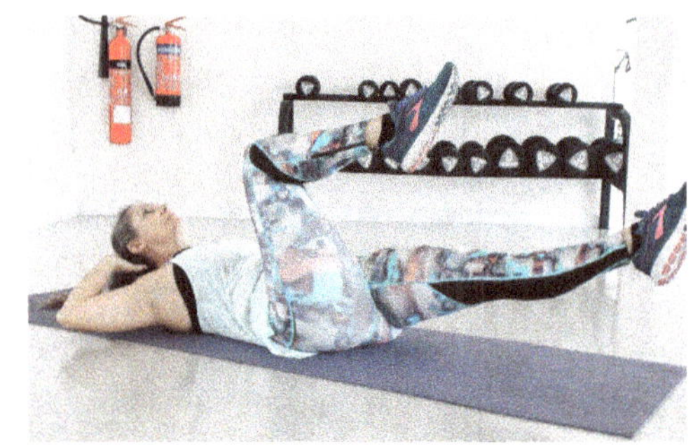

CORE: STABILITY AND MOBILITY STRENGTH

Working on your core strength will help you to move pain-free through menopause and well after that. As I am writing this updated version of my ST guide (first edition 2017) I am sitting in an elastic back brace. UGH. How did I get myself into this physical position?

Well number one, and this is very important to know is that I am, like the rest of you, a human. I am almost 54 years old and at risk of deterioration, injury, weight gain and illness just like everyone else. In 2022, I was sick most of the year. I coughed for an entire year, had bronchitis twice, had awful flu during the summer, then was put on a nebuliser and stronger asthma meds and by December I caught Influenza A and pneumonia. Double whammy for the holidays. Without going into massive detail, I ended going to see a Chinese doctor, and had 7 sessions of acupuncture with a "hot box" over my lungs, some cupping and she also bled my ears (from the top lobe, weird!). I had three sessions of her specially brewed tea, which I drank hot three times a day.

Come today, which is now February 2023, I am no longer coughing. I am also off all Pharma, no steroids, no inhalers. Feeling fab.

What did I do as soon as I felt better? I went back to triathlon training, resumed my online kettlebell classes like a blooming hero and during a push plank jump my back gave a very loud CLACK.

So, here's a lesson from me. If you have been off training for a while, start from the bottom up. Literally.

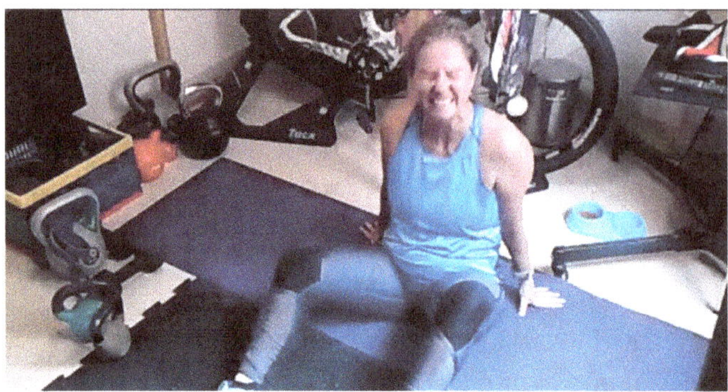

See this image?

That is me during that kettlebell class. I couldn't get up. I was immobilised! I had to call my husband and I also have a screenshot of the faces of my two clients with their jaw dropped. I laugh now... but.

So, when I say start from the bottom up, I mean work on your core first before attempting your regular long rides or runs. Or your heavy kettlebell swings. Get a grip on your core, work at it, strengthen it, or you will possibly end up where I am sitting now.

We (women) generate most of our strength and stability through our hips. We tend to have powerful lower body muscles, but our core is weak. That's why I could go out and bash out a 65km ride after two months of inactivity, but then feel a crippling lower back pain afterwards.

It's time to build glute, hip and core strength. If you don't, you can set yourself up for ligament tears and other orthopaedic issues. Women in menopause with weak core muscles can also suffer from incontinence. So, let's listen to sports physiologists and start from the ground up.

Yep, that is the cat's bowl behind me. We share the room. I should charge him rent.

- Sit Up
- Hip Abduction on Mat
- Hip Adduction on Mat
- Spinal Twist with leg over
- Hamstring Curl with Ball
- Plank (front and side)
- Plank with Knee Dip
- Side Reaches on Mat
- Bird Dog
- Abdominal Crunches
- Hip Lifts

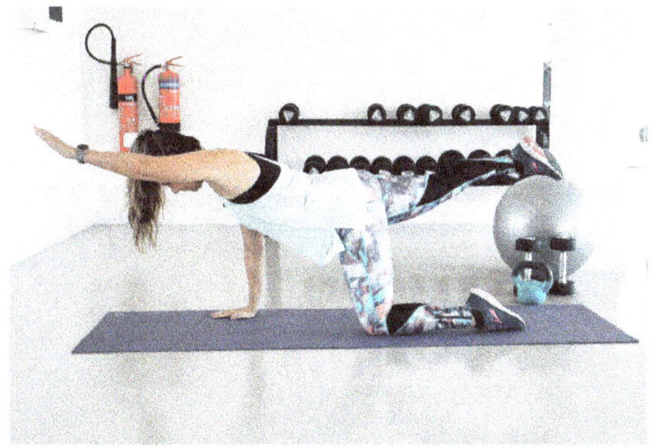

SIT UP

Lie down and squeeze the small of your back into the floor. Feet flat on the floor, fingers behind your ears. Sit up, trying to keep a "hip hinge" position and a straight back. Return.

If you have difficulty keeping your feet on the floor, you can hook them under the sofa or a bench, depending on where you are working out.

HIP ABDUCTION ON MAT

These abduction exercises, engage the TFL (tensor fasciae latae) and help strengthen the hip joint.

Start on your side, with one foot behind the other. Make sure the hips are facing forwards and not rocking back, and your start and finish position is with your foot behind the bottom leg. Raise your leg up and down, and make sure that you keep your hips facing the opposite wall. Do not allow your foot to collapse behind you, ease it down.

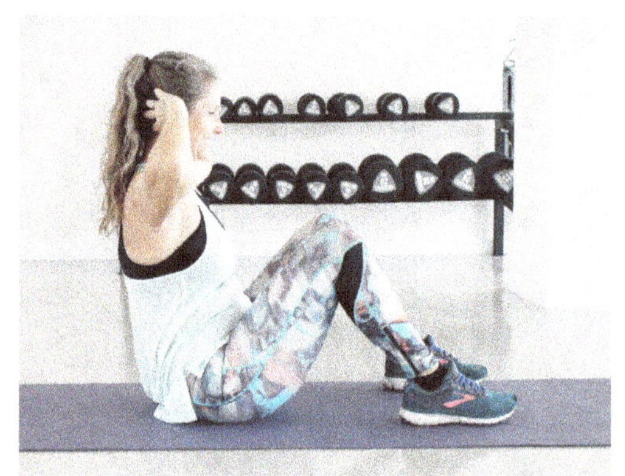

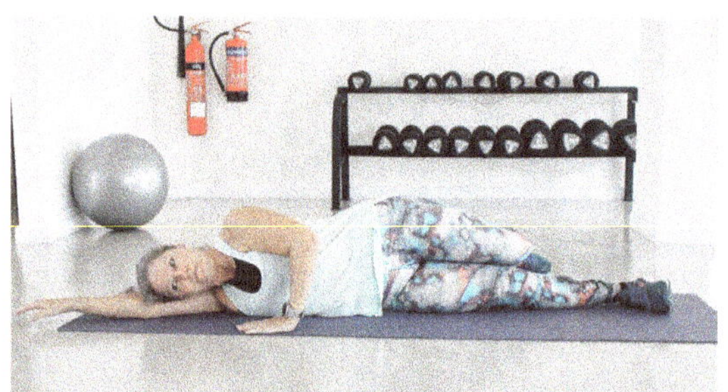

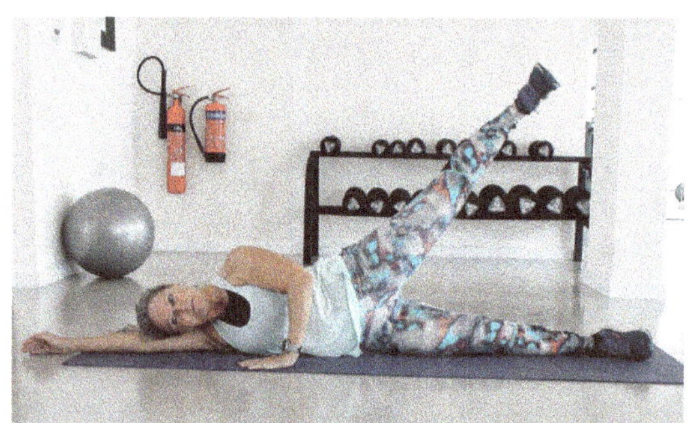

"As seen with Jane Fonda 1982"

HIP ADDUCTION ON MAT

Now to work the hip adductors, where you will raise the lower leg with a flexed foot. Keep the top leg behind your knee while you are lifting.

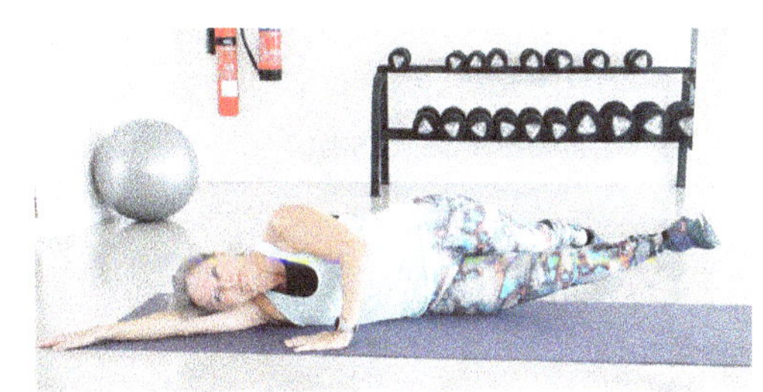

SPINAL TWIST

This exercise uses core strength and engages your oblique muscles.

Be sure to keep your shoulder blades to the floor as best you can, keep your feet together and do not allow them to collapse to the floor. Ease them down slowly. Repeat each side.

Press the small of your back into the floor, raise your legs keeping knees slightly bend.

Twist the lower body right to left, slowly. Don't allow the feet to crash to the floor and keep your knees and feet close together.

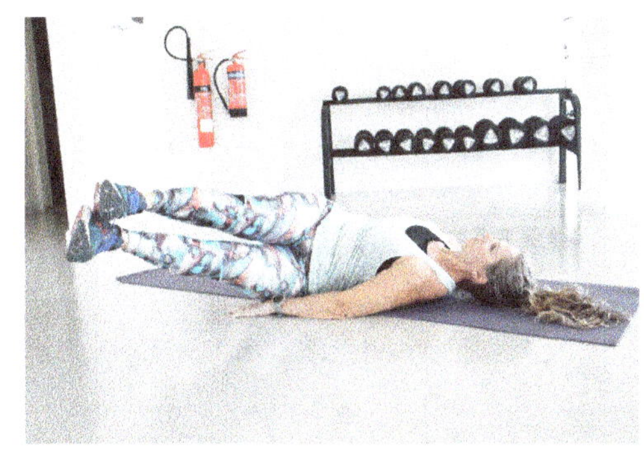

HAMSTRING CURL

Lie flat and centre your feet almost hip width apart on the ball.

Lift the hips and engage the core, drawing the ball towards you.

Roll out your legs away and draw in again.

Try not to drop the hips while extending and flexing the knee joint.

PLANKS (FRONT AND SIDE)

With planks, it's important to be aware where your hip position is, and not rock backwards or forwards. The hips need to be "open". Make sure your chest is facing forwards too, and that you don't have a saggy bottom. *(You can also rest your elbow on your stability disc for this, it's really comfortable).*

In the photo below you can see that my hips need to come down a bit for an improved plank position. Keep your elbows under your shoulders and try relax the neck. Easier said than done.

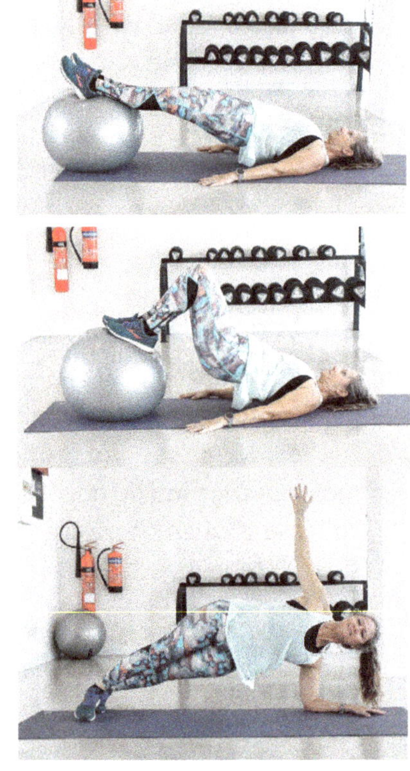

Nobody wants a saggy bottom!

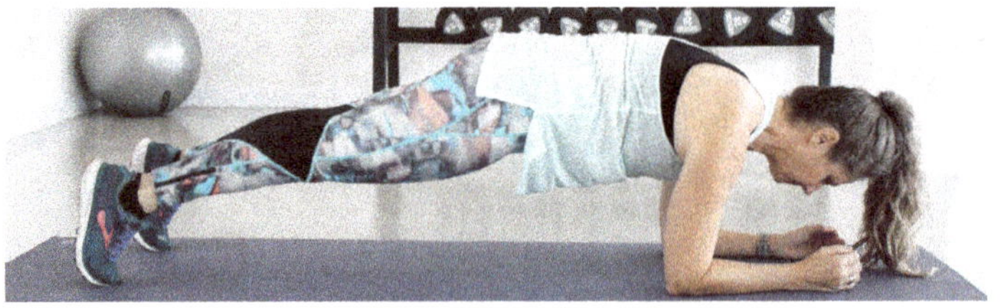

PLANK WITH KNEE DIP

From a forearm plank position, draw in the knee and alternate sides.

Try a variation of this knee dip, by planking on your hands. Again, as with all planks, keep your shoulder over your hands.

If you have two stability balls, try resting one hand on each one.

SIDE REACHES

Engage the core and left your shoulder blades, reach down each side of your body and return.

Try to reach your foot, keeping the core tight and shoulder blades off the floor.

BIRD DOG

With practice, bird dogs strengthen the muscles around your joints, improving mobility in your arms and legs. They can also relieve lower back pain and they are really a whole-body engagement exercise. Make sure your middle is not sagging to the floor and you are pulling up the core to seek a tabletop back.

Alternate this position each side.

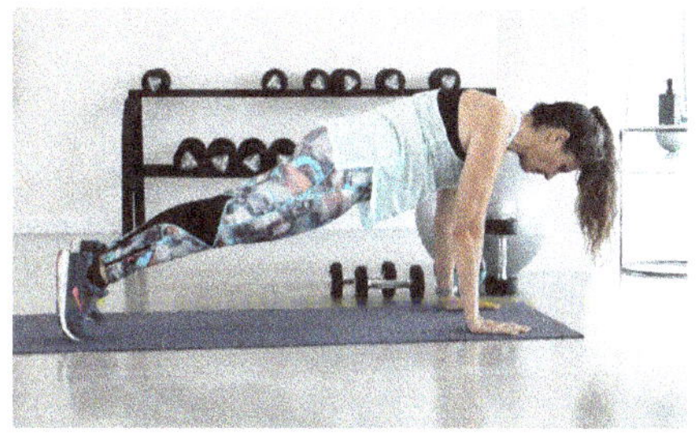

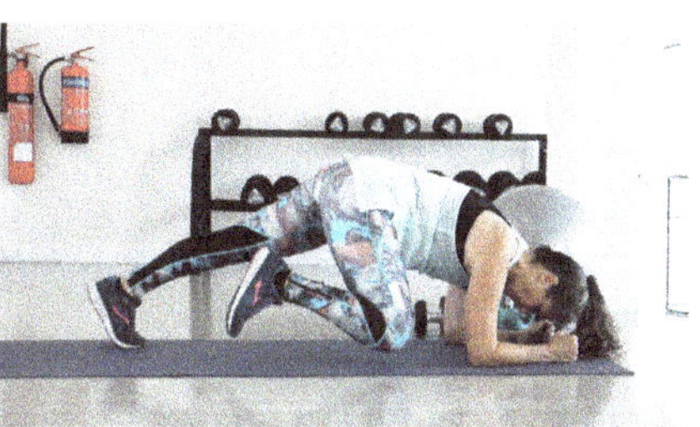

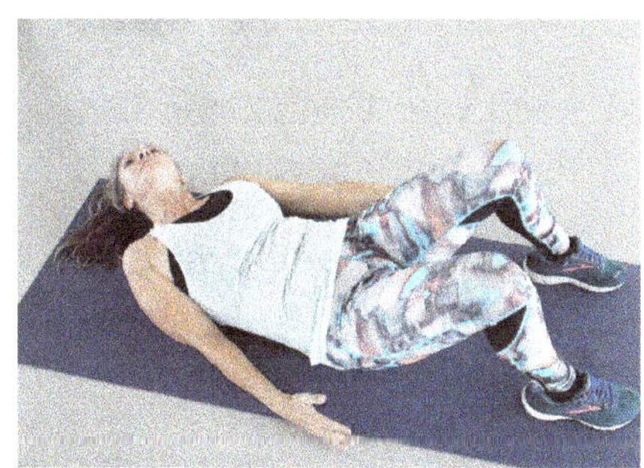

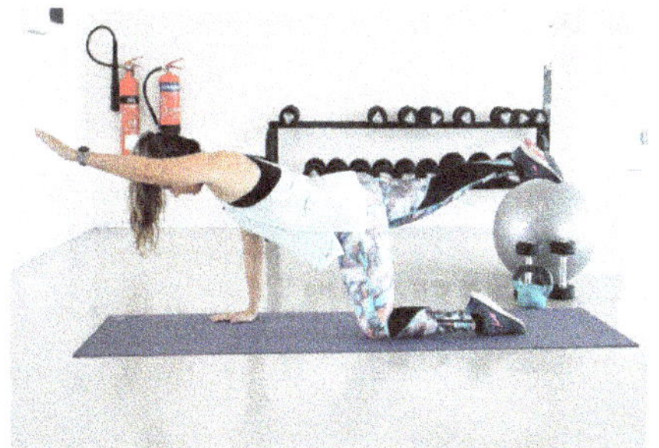

CRUNCHES

Good old-fashioned crunches!

Again, keep your lower back squeezed to the floor, raise the shoulder blades and "crunch" the elbows towards the knees. Keep the shoulder blades off the floor for all the designated repetitions.

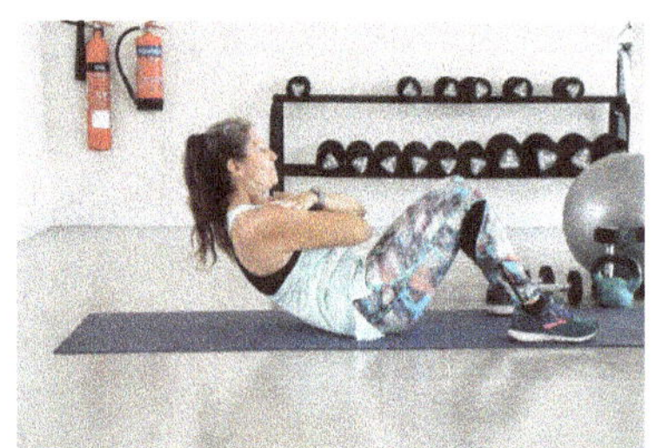

Try crossing your arms over your chest too for a variation.

REVERSE CRUNCH

Lift your feet off the ground and raise your thighs until they're vertical.

Keep your knees bent at 90 degrees throughout the movement.

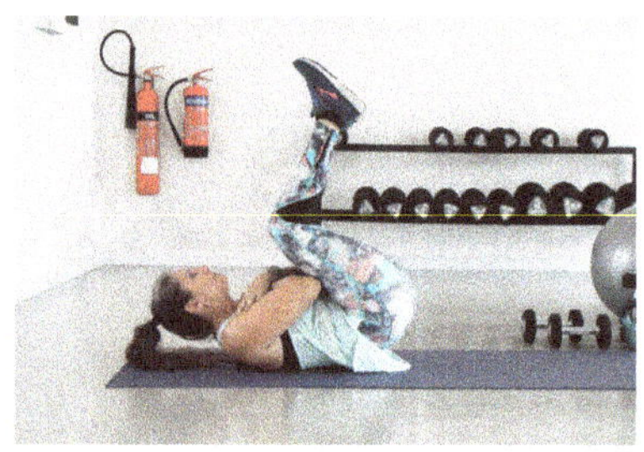

Tuck your knees toward your face as far as you can comfortably go without lifting your mid-back from the mat.

Your hips and lower back should lift off the ground.

HIP LIFTS

Rather like a reverse crunch, lift your feet off the ground and raise your legs until vertical. Keep your knees soft. Lift your hips without lifting your mid-back from the mat.

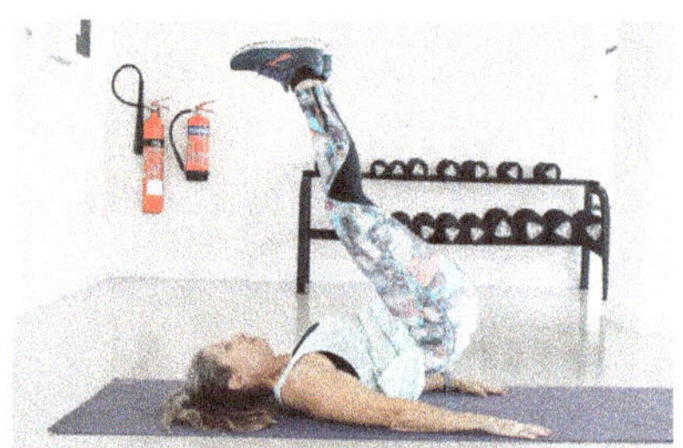

Use your abs to lift, not your back! Slow movement up and down.

In this last piece, before I go into some ideas on how to do SIT, I want to cover a few basic upper body exercises. Whether you're a swimmer, cyclist, runner or triathlete, or just wanting to attack your "guns", you need to train your upper body. Your upper body needs strengthening to avoid compensation in your lower back, especially if you are a triathlete on aero bars.

The following exercises are generic, and you will probably find them in most endurance training programmes. My preference is always my kettlebell sequences, but if you don't have access to kettlebells these exercises will be equally as beneficial, using bodyweight and dumbbells.

1.   Renegade Row

2.   Bicep Curl

3.   Chest Press on Ball or Bench

4.   Arm Raise with Dumbbell

5.   Dumbbell Pullover on Ball

6.   Triceps Extension

7.   Single Arm Row with Ball or Bench

8.   Push Ups

You will need a set of dumbbells, a bench, a mat and your well-pumped exercise ball.

RENEGADE ROW

It is best to use hex dumbbells with a flat side to rest on as the round dumbbells may roll under the inexperienced. This gym in particular only has round dumbbells, so I balanced my other arm on my closed fist, as I kept rolling out and collapsing. Ah well.

Row the weight upward until your upper arm is higher than your torso, then slowly lower it back down to the ground.

Add a knee dip for variation.

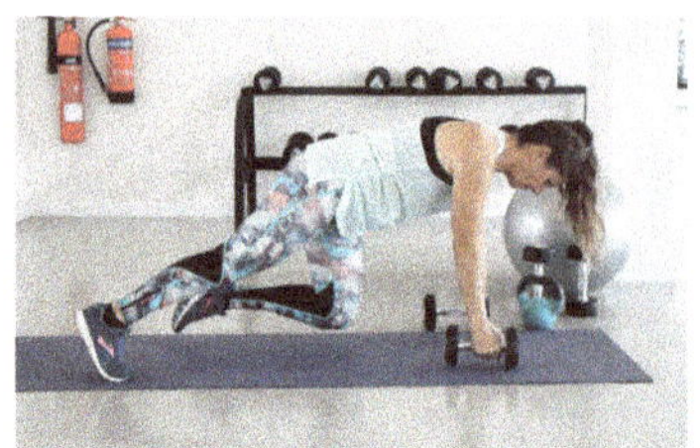

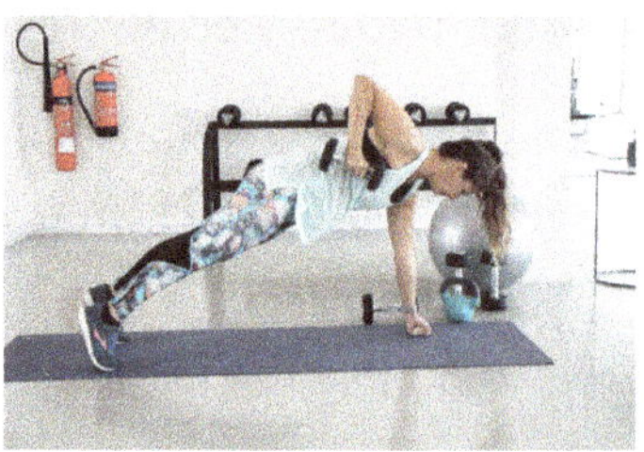

BICEP CURL

Stand tall, feet under hips, core engaged. With straight arms by your side, hold the dumbbells firmly and raise them upwards, return to side.

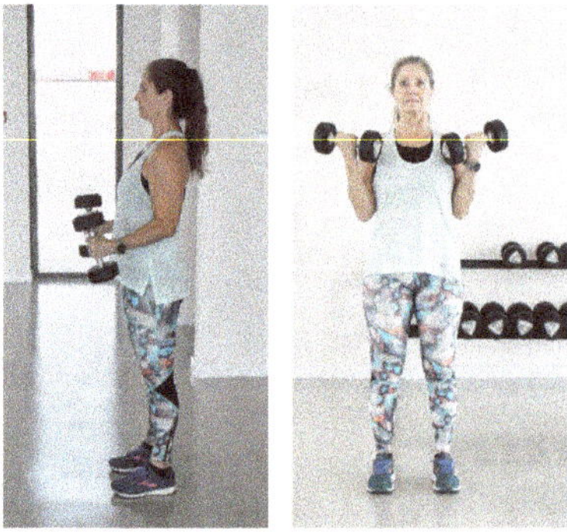

CHEST PRESS ON BALL OR BENCH

Centre your back on the ball but your neck should be supported.

Bridge the hips. Push the dumbbells up and lower down slowly. They should be aligned with your chest.

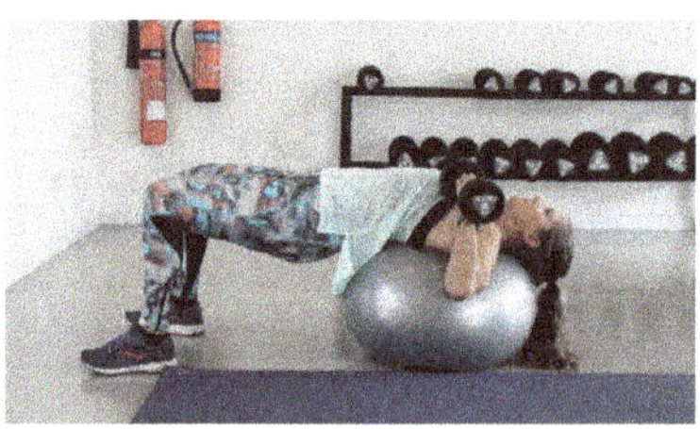

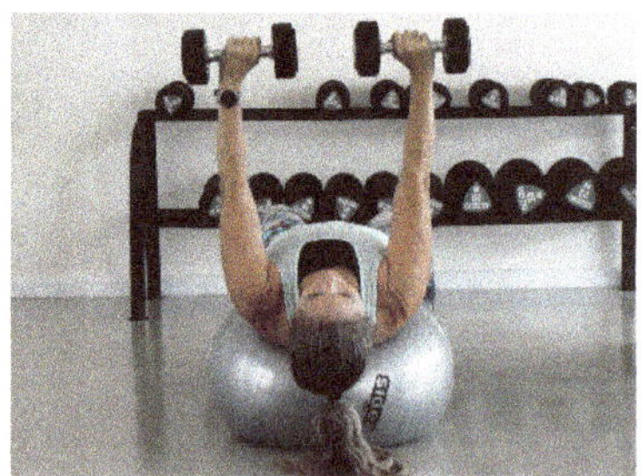

ARM RAISE WITH DUMBBELL

Standing in the same position as you would for the bicep curl, raise the arms up and down slowly keeping the arms straight.

Keep the core engaged.

DUMBBELL PULLOVER ON BALL

Place your shoulder blades on the ball, bridge the hips. Hold the end of the dumbbell (or a kettlebell) and raise above your face. Then lower the arms backwards over your head keeping them straight, and return.

TRICEPS EXTENSION

In a split squat position, keep the arm aligned with your body when extending the dumbbell backwards.

You should feel this effort in your upper arm at the back (triceps).

Extend the arm backwards as best you can and return to the starting position.

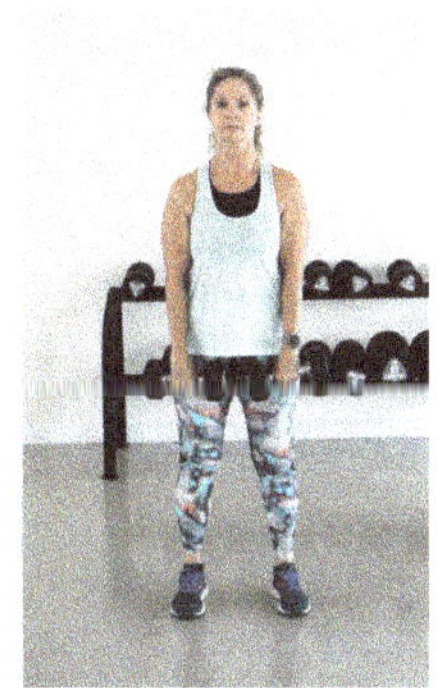
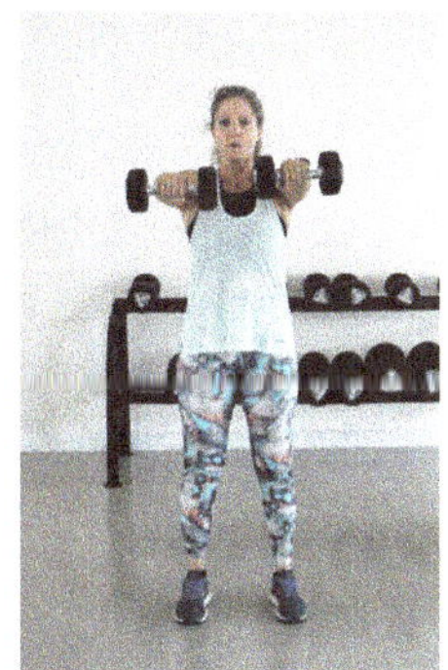

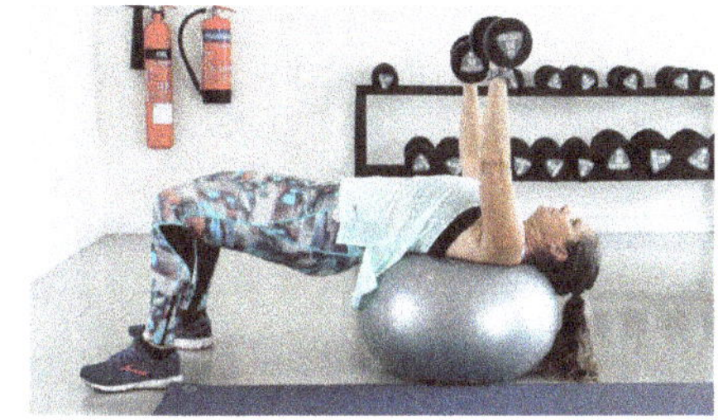

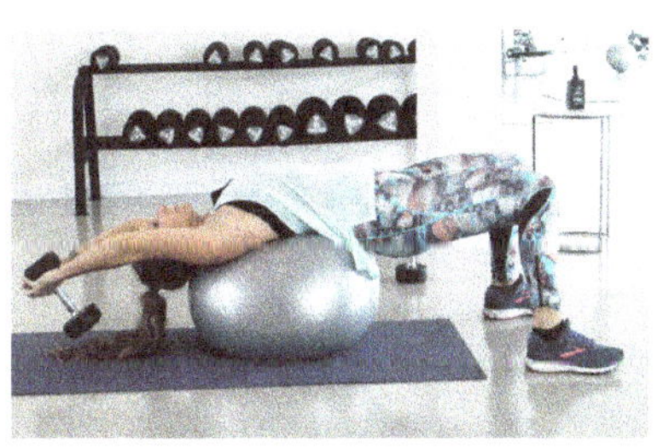

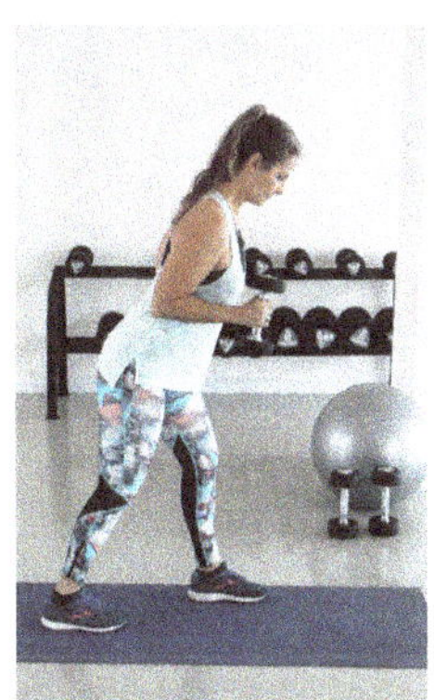
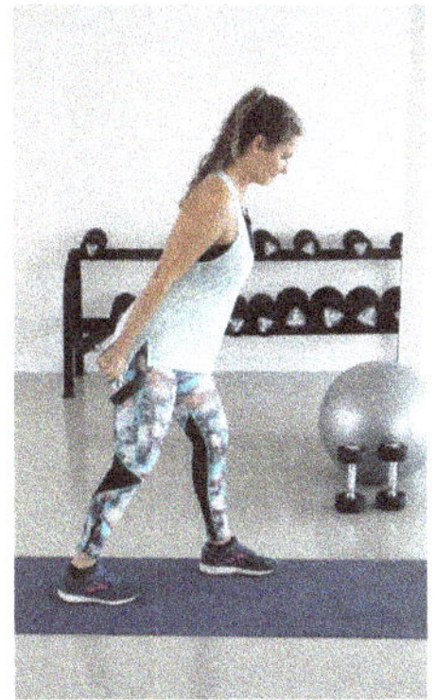

SINGLE ARM ROW WITH BALL OR BENCH

Resting your knee on a ball or bench, keeping a tabletop back, row the dumbbell.

Keep your elbow close to your body.

PUSH UPS

At the time of going to press, the press-up demonstration photo was not taken (I forgot, even with a checklist), so I've had to take one from my Zoom class videos.

Your start position should be with your hands underneath your shoulders, spread your fingers until and have your feet hip width apart. Lower yourself as much as you can without (again), a saggy bottom. We are trying to avoid saggy bottoms, after all.

It doesn't matter if you find this hard. *Start with one push-up. One. And tomorrow, do two.*

And so, it starts. You're doing great!!!

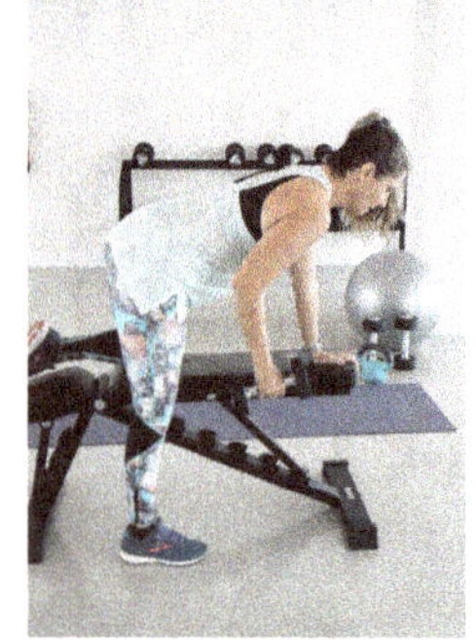
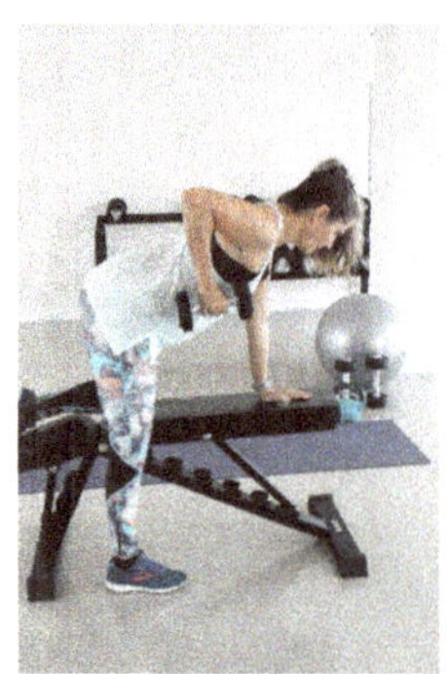
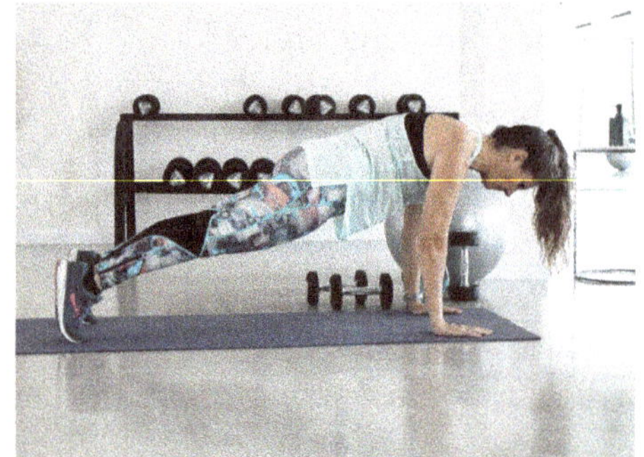
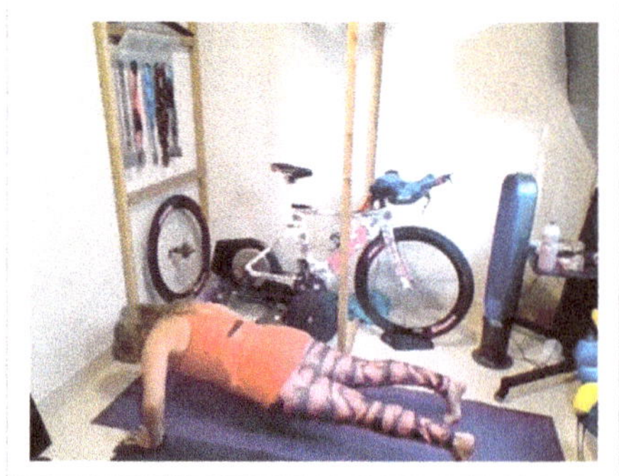

PLYOMETRICS AND "SIT"

Plyometrics work gives your bones and muscles the extra stimulus that comes when you push off against gravity and land back down. Plyometric work is essential to women in perimenopause and menopause because this technique works on their explosive power and muscle integrity, for those fast-firing muscles (sprints), and to maintain that fast twitch and that neuromuscular stimulation for a strong, fast contraction.

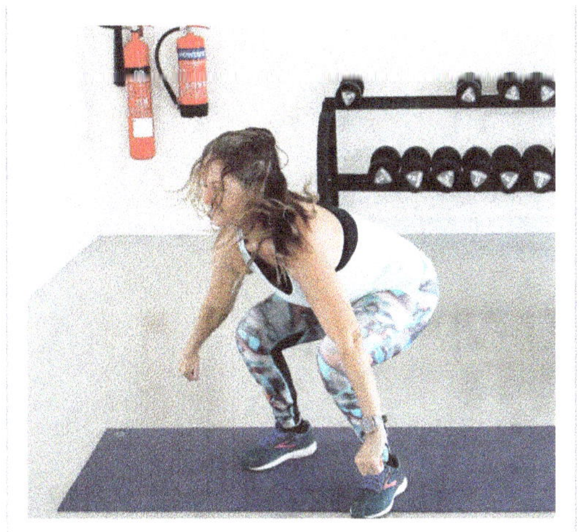

Over the past decade, it has been convincingly shown that performing repeated brief supramaximal cycle sprints regularly (i.e. sprint interval training [SIT]), is associated with aerobic adaptations and health benefits similar to or greater than with moderate-intensity continuous training (MICT). So, you do not always have to do "LSD" rides and runs (long and slow), you can get amazing and effective training done in just 30 minutes.

Let's start off with some basic plyometric moves and then see how it all hangs together with some SIT ideas. Remember that with SIT, the key is to not overdo it. Generally, two sessions a week are enough combined in with your other planned training, but in peak season when you are racing or training a lot then one session a week should suffice.

TOP TIP: if you have long hair, tie it up!

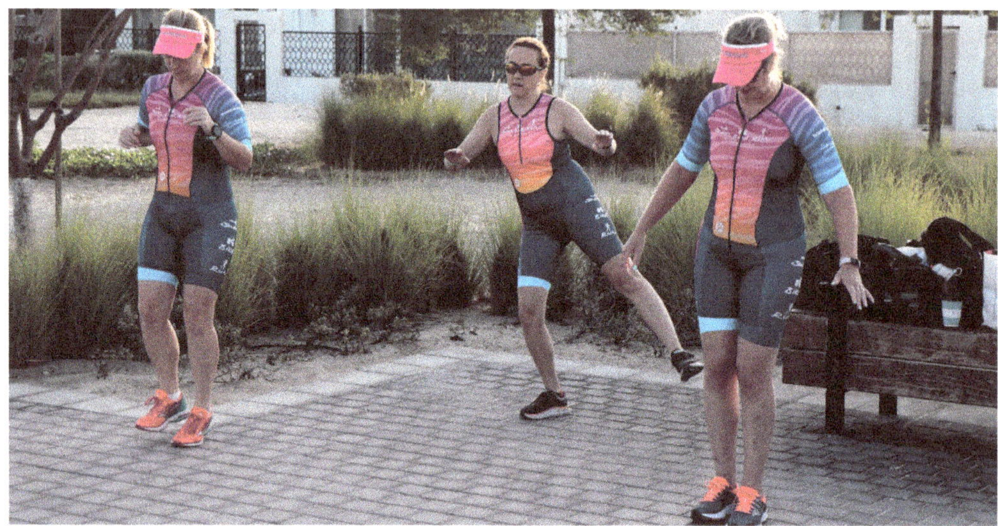

SIT is often promoted as a time-efficient exercise strategy, and the most studied SIT protocol (*4-6 repeated 30-s Wingate sprints with 4 min recovery, here referred to as 'classic' SIT*) takes up to approximately 30 min per session. (The Wingate test is a 30-second, all-out sprint on a stationary cycle against a braking torque).

It is those impacts, big or small, that generate important physiological changes. You are essentially training your muscles to detonate on-demand and explosively. If you're racing, think of sprint finishes, if you're out on a group ride, a breakaway or catching on the group in front of you. You will be able to apply the strength you gain through SIT to gain speed. Remember, this is where you get the benefits—improved insulin sensitivity, stronger mitochondria, improved fat burning (especially deep visceral fat), and an ever-important boost of growth hormone after you finish!

Imagine, 30 minutes is all you need!

You will need a mat, a set of kettlebells, and your own great body for the bodyweight stuff.

Exercise physiologist Dr Stacy Sims recommends that during your off-season, when you're not out running, riding, hiking, or doing big events, you do up to three SIT workouts a week, so long as you allow your body ample recovery time to bounce back week to week. If you are currently training (for an event/race), then just one or two sessions a week is ample.

BODYWEIGHT PLYOMETRIC EXERCISES

1.   Tuck Jump

2.   Depth Jump

3.   Squat Jump

4.   Plyo Jumps

5.   Heiden Jumps

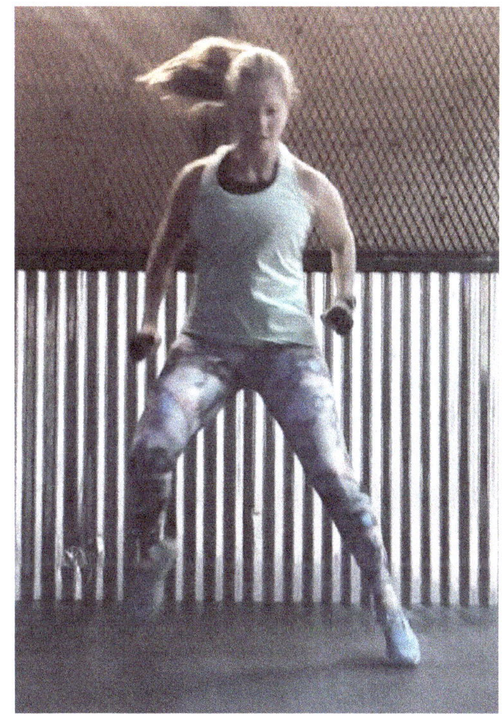

Warning for MENO BODS: air or pee can escape during plyometrics.

"No Need To Apologise......"

TUCK JUMP

Start by standing with your feet a little less than shoulder-width apart. Drop down a little into a quarter squat then explode into the air. Keep your back straight throughout and tuck your knees up towards your chest as much as possible, before landing as softly as you can, keeping your feet, knees and hips in alignment as you land.

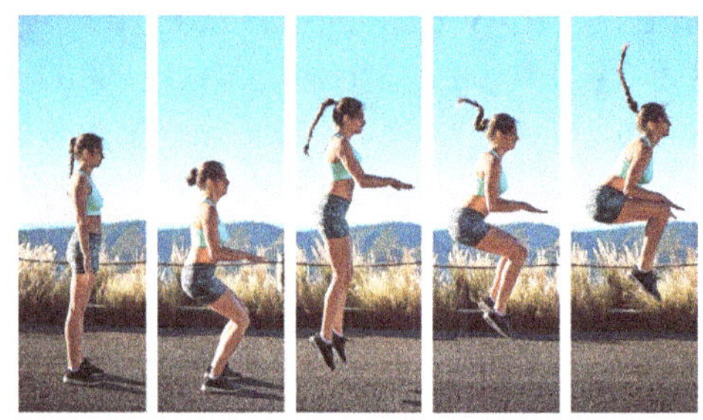

PANTHERMEDIAGMBH/ALAMYSTOCKPHOTO

DEPTH JUMP

This exercise trains the ability to absorb force and utilize elastic energy to produce greater concentric muscular force. Stand at the front edge of a box or bench.

Step up to it. Then jump off, and land on two feet. (if you have an ankle injury, do not do this exercise until you have consulted with your physio).

SQUAT JUMP

Stand with your feet just outside shoulder- width apart, toes pointed in front (mine are slightly outward, that is my limitation). Squat down with your weight in your heels, chest up, knees over toes, and a neutral spine.

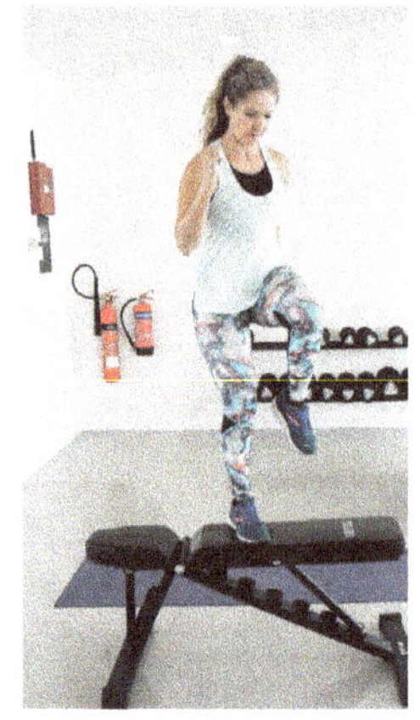

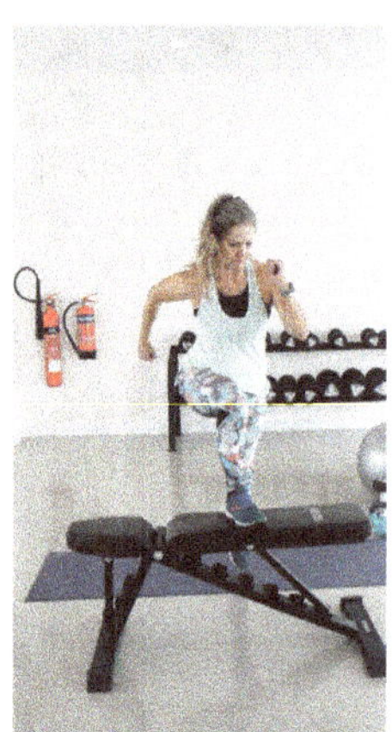

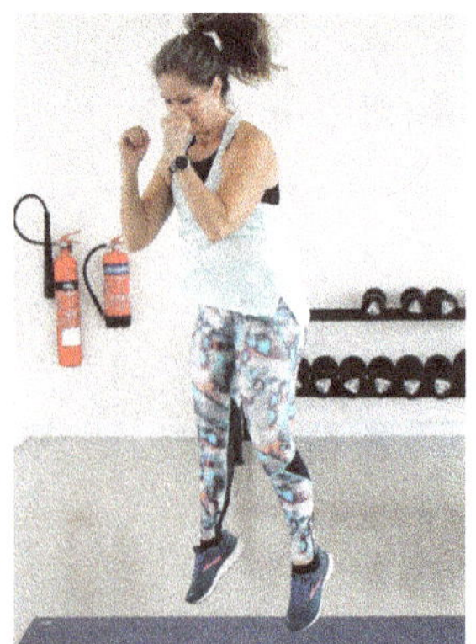

When you hit the bottom of your squat, squeeze your butt tight and drive hard through your legs and heels as you launch straight up, pushing off your toes at the last moment of contact with the floor.

Then use the momentum from landing to go right into your next squat.

PLYO SPLIT SQUAT JUMPS

Stand upright with your feet together and your arms at your side.

Jump in the air and land in a split squat position so that your right leg is forward with the knee bent and your left leg is backward standing on your toes.

Without pausing, jump in the air again and reverse the position of your legs.

Perform for 30- to 60-second intervals.

HEIDEN JUMPS (LATERAL BOUNDING)

With feet hip-width apart, bend your knees to squat straight down. Keep your weight on your heels. Shift weight from heels to toes as you begin your jump, quickly push upward and sideways toward the other side of the line. Land softly and absorb the shock by squatting deeply. Repeat.

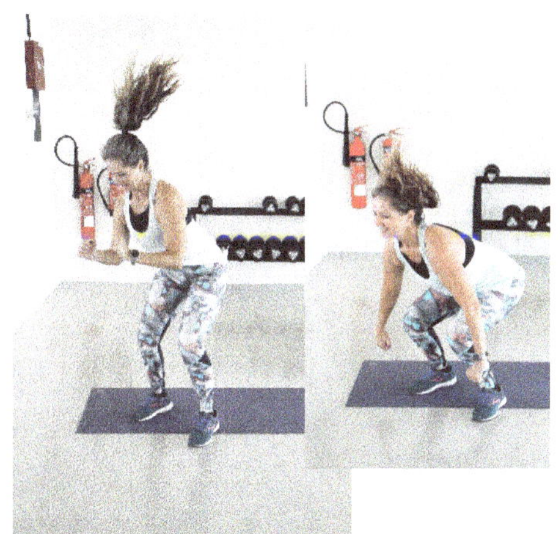

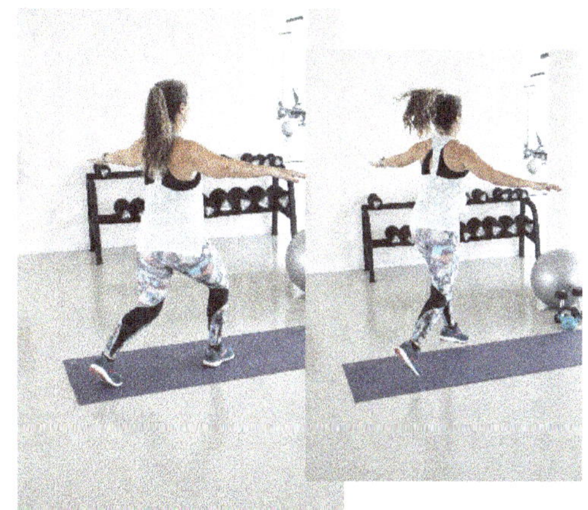

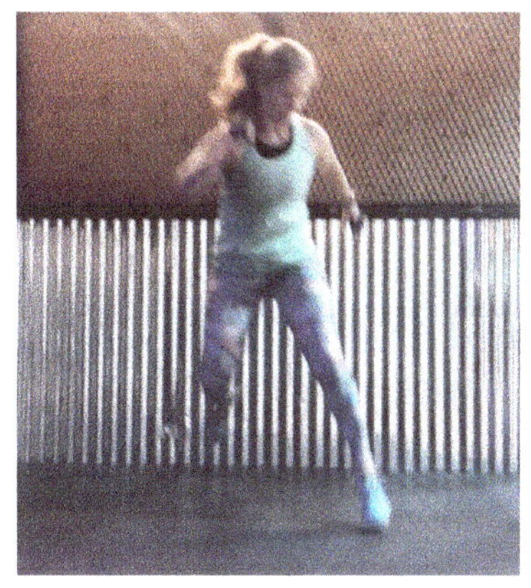

SIT – LET'S PUT IT ALL TOGETHER

So you now have a stack of exercises that you can combine into a workout. But how?

Here are some ideas below. Remember, you only really need 30 minutes of workout time, and then spend some time before and after stretching and doing dynamic warm up. The "hard part" in between the warmup and cool down need only be 15/20 minutes (INTENSE!)

For the warm-up, use your band for band walks and the hip flexor warmer, stability disc, a broomstick (!), and you can use small kettlebells or dumbbells to start your movement.

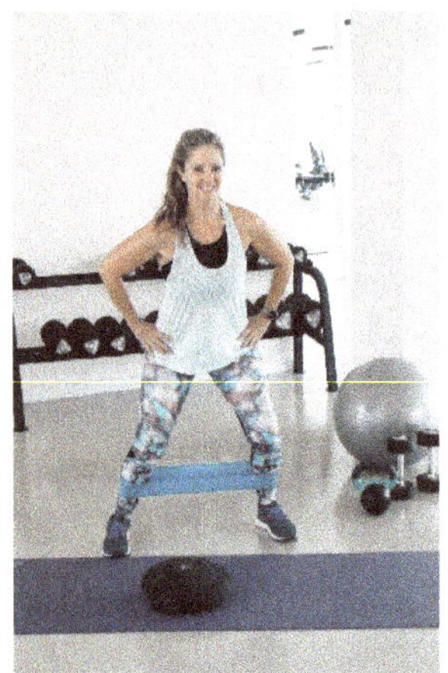
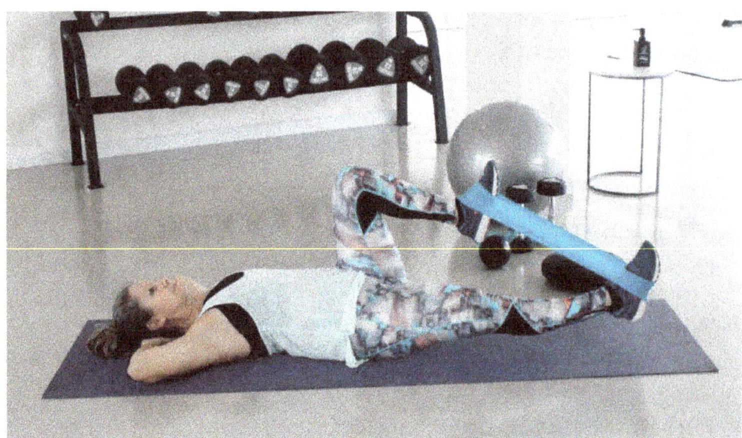

Do hip openers in the 90/90 position (remember the MEAUXTION channel I spoke of earlier). Inchworms, bird dogs, glute bridging, use the roller, do deadlifts with a light weight, going into some lightweight swings, halos and slingshots. (Kettlebell Kings have loads of movements online for you to look at).

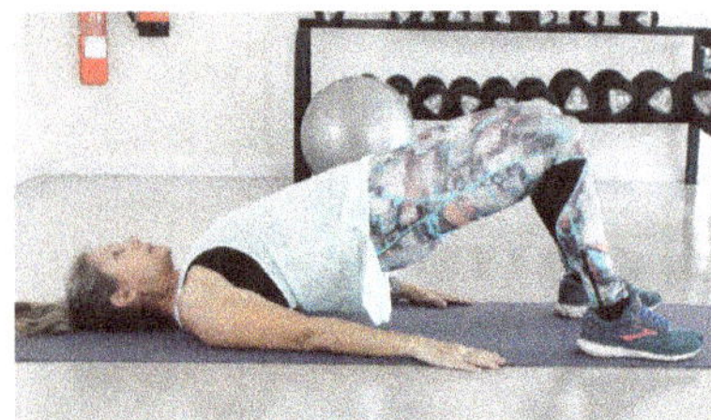
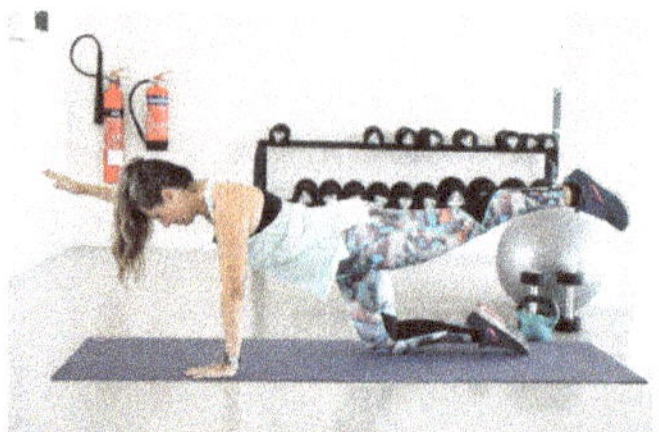
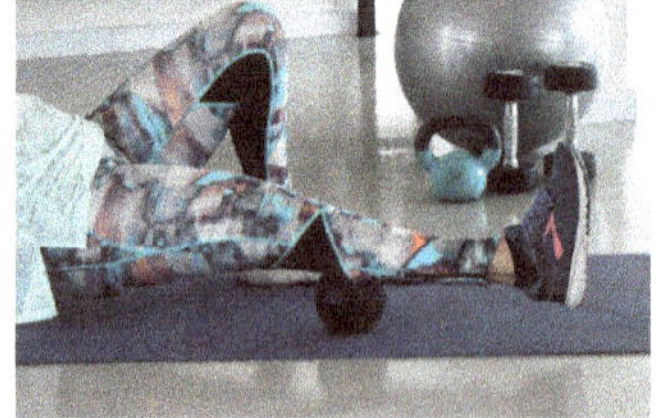

WORKOUT ONE

Try to do up to six rounds of this plyometric workout. Put in some jump squats, Heiden Jumps, skipping, body weight push-ups and even some V-ups or sit-ups. You could add in some burpees or push plank jumps and then a shuttle sprint. (It should be 4 exercises, shuttle run, then rest.)

Set your interval timer (downloadable to your phone from the internet), each "pack" of exercises should be about 4 minutes.

20 jump squats.

Then as you roll into the second minute, do 40 jumping jacks or skipping.

Then you roll into the next one, do 10 push-ups to side planks.

Then roll into V-ups or sit-ups and do 10 Once you've done these, do a shuttle run down the corridor until your 4 minutes beep.

Then rest for one minute and start again. Try two rounds and work up to six rounds.

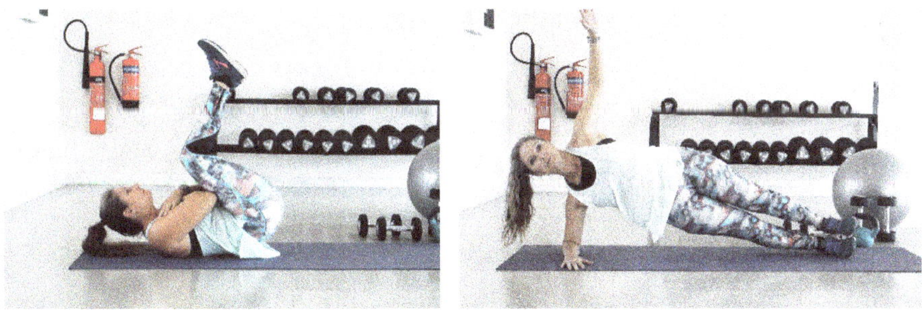

This is a way to encompass both high intensity and plyo work, in a total of 42 minutes if you do six rounds. Variation, add in kettlebell swings!

WORKOUT TWO

This is a "Kettlebell Burner". Try five to eight rounds. Do your warmup as above, and you can also use a rowing machine, indoor bike or treadmill for 5 minutes however the warm-up exercises must be done to help with your mobility.

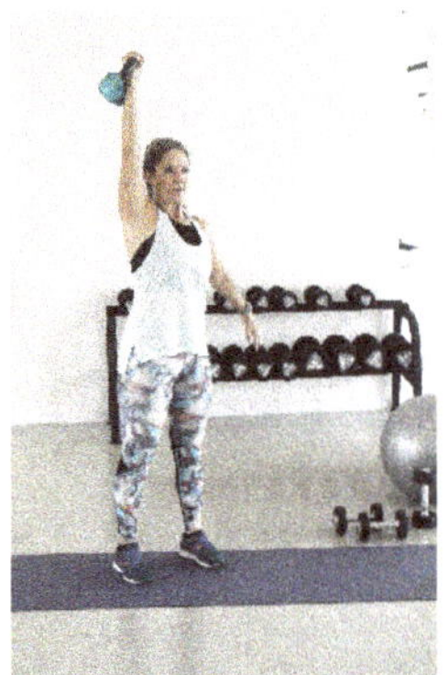 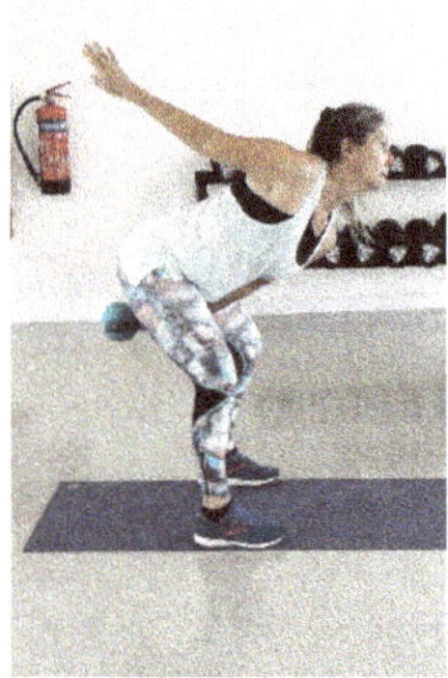 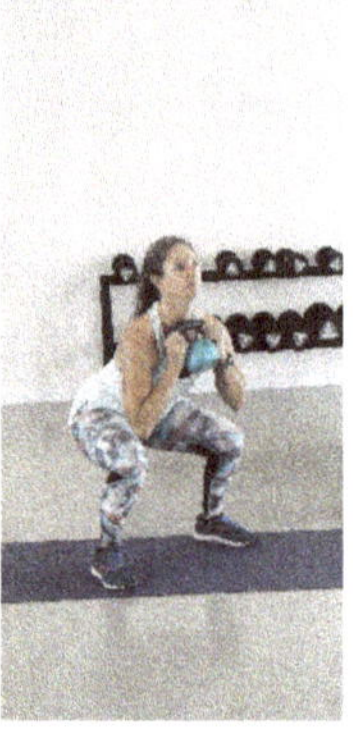 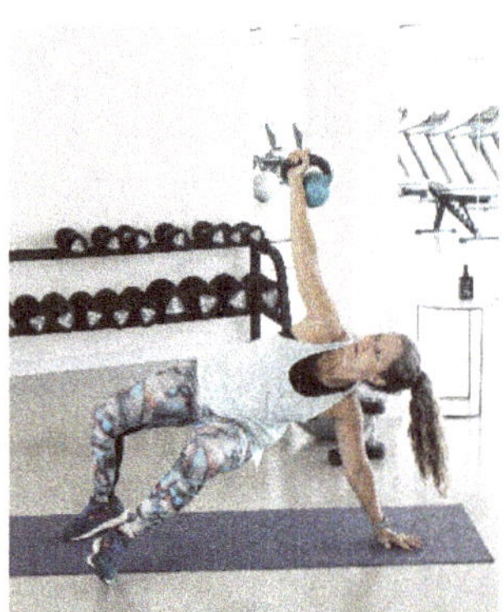

Not all of these movements are in this manual (there are so many!) so you can use a reliable source to check the correct posture and movement. (My personal favourite is kettlebell champion Brittany van Schravendijk as a reference.

- 10 x kettlebell bell single arm swing
- 10 x kettlebell clean and overhead press
- 10 x kettlebell goblet squats
- 10 trunk twists with a light bar or broomstick
- 10 Turkish-Getups (5 each side with Kettlebell)
- Finish off with planks, 5 x 20 seconds on, 10 seconds off.

Cool down with some mobility and recovery.

WORKOUT THREE

Try this "SIT" workout doing 1 minute on.... 20 seconds off.
Play with it.

It's a 30-minute workout and aim for 5 rounds.

Always, always, do your mobility and warm- up first.

Then:

5-10 deadlifts - you can use a barbell or kettlebell or dumbbells for this (if you stand on the bottom step of the staircase, you get a little more reach...)

20 step-ups (bench, your patio, your step) 12 burpees or push-plank-jumps

10 push-ups

14 squats or reverse lunge

20 tuck jumps or high knees (like height skipping)

Do your mobility to finish. (Try not to look like a rabbit's eyes in the headlights when you do your tuck jump!)

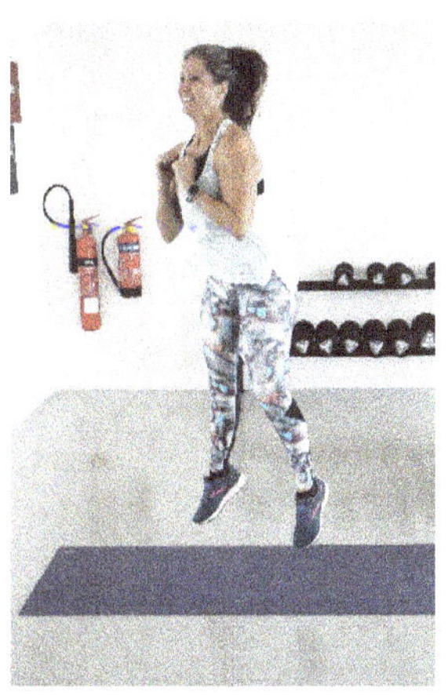

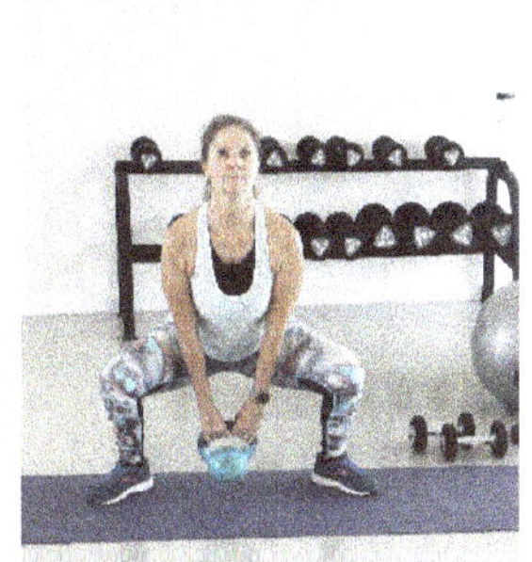

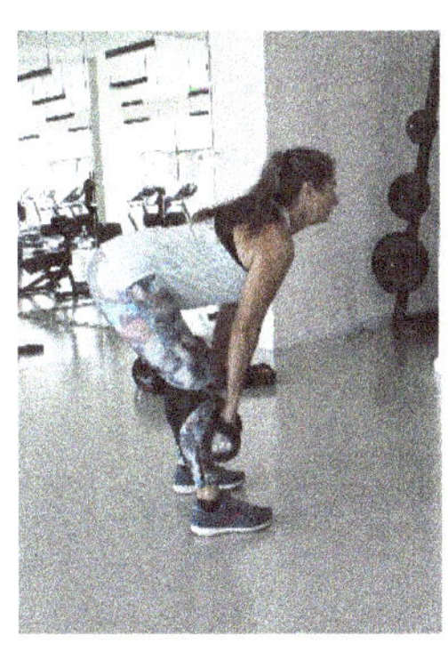

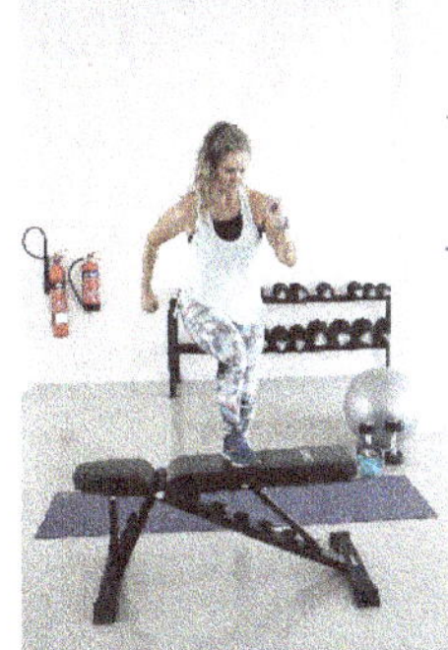

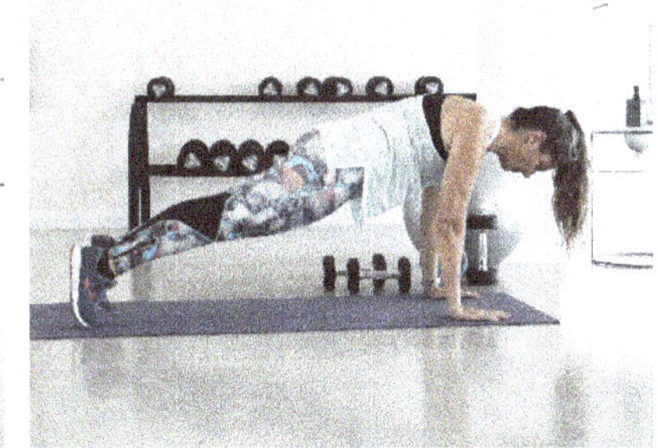

WORKOUT FOUR

Traditionally, a SIT workout is 7 minutes, and remember, strengthening the body now determines quality of life later in life. (Credit for this workout is the Greatist website.)

See how effective this workout is, that you could do it as an active rest day (if you are so inclined, or, add it to a "3-a-day" training plan for example, do the SIT in the morning before work, your yoga and stretching midday and a nice easy run in the evening.

Always, do your mobility and warm-up first for 10 to 15 minutes (rolling, band work etc)

Then start your 7 minutes:

Perform each exercise below at a high-intensity effort for 30 seconds. For static exercises such as the wall sit and plank, hold the position for 30 seconds. For exercises that target two sides (such as your legs), alternate sides for 30 seconds. Rest for 5 seconds after each exercise.

Make this list, write it on your board, and get on it.

Jumping jacks, Wall sit (you can use your exercise ball), Push-up, Crunch, Step-up, Squat, Tricep dip, Plank, Jump Squat, Lunge, Push-up with Rotation, Side plank. Repeat from the top and stop after 7 minutes. How many rounds did you get?

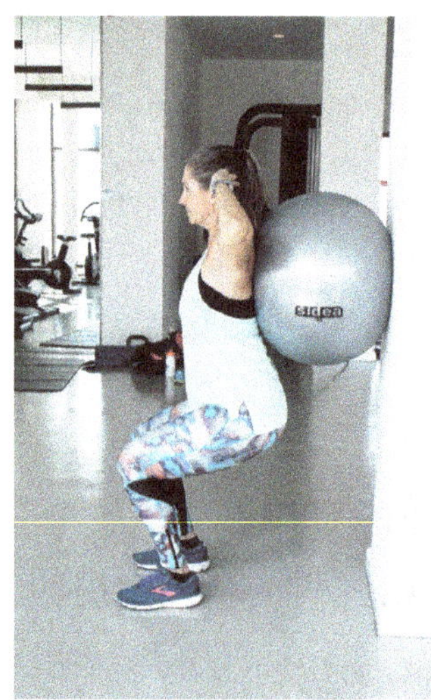

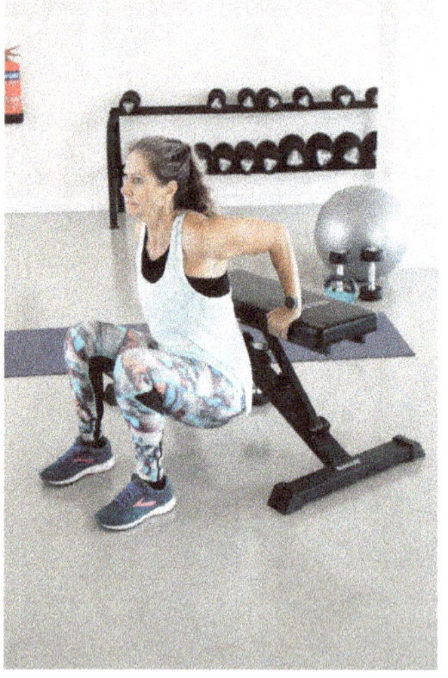

WORKOUT FIVE

The objective of this training set is to give you a block of high intensity and a short recovery and repeat. It is more of a traditional HITT set, rather than the 7-minute SIT.

Programme yourself 6 rounds of Kettlebell swings of 2 minute efforts, 100-metre run or row in between.

Warm up and warm down either end by either running or rowing, and do the mobility sequence, always!

When you run, put a smile on! Why?

It is proven, and hear me out here, that smiling when exercising increases time to fatigue. Seriously! .

Researchers at Ulster University and Swansea University asked a group of 24 runners to wear a breathing mask to measure oxygen consumption and then complete four six-minute running blocks on a treadmill while smiling or frowning. The study, which was recently published in Psychology of Sport and Exercise, found that runners who smiled used less oxygen, ran more economically and had a lower perceived rate of exertion than those who frowned and those in the control group.

So get swinging, and get smiling!

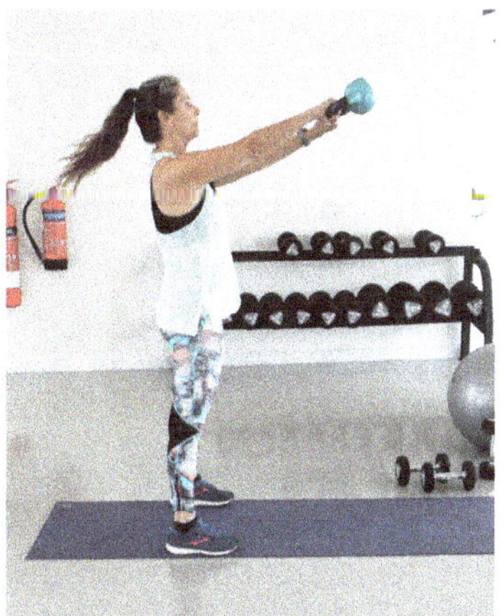

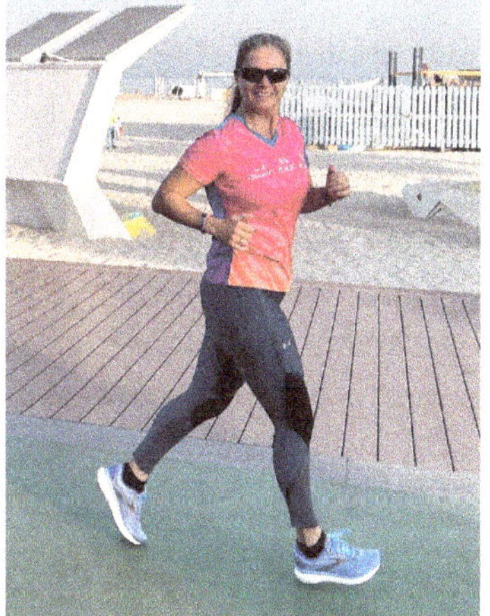

STRETCHING AND FLEXIBILITY

After you have finished your workouts, spend some time taking care of your muscles.

Get down into a **PIGEON POSE**. From all fours, bring your right knee forward towards your right wrist. Experiment with what feels right for you, giving you a stretch on your outer hip without any discomfort in your knee.

Slide your left leg back and point your toes, your heel is pointing up to the ceiling. Scissor your hips together, by drawing your legs in towards each other. Use some support under your right buttock if needed, to keep your hips level. As you inhale, come onto your fingertips, lengthen your spine, draw your navel in and open your chest.

As you exhale, walk your hands forward and lower your upper body towards the floor. You can rest your forearms and forehead on the mat.

Then do a **HIP FLEXOR STRETCH** (especially if you sit a long time for work). Kneel on your leg and bend your other leg out in front of you, with that foot flat on the floor.

Keeping your back straight, slowly push your hips forward until you feel a stretch in the upper thigh of your back leg and hip. Place your hands on the floor and lift them up one at a time to open the thoracic cavity and stretch. Hold the stretch for at least 15 to 30 seconds.

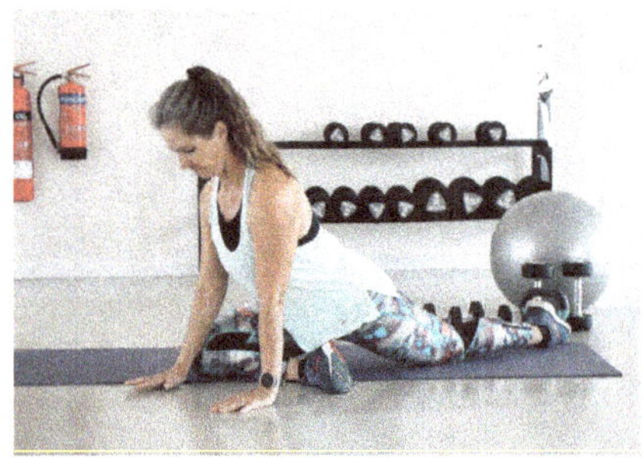

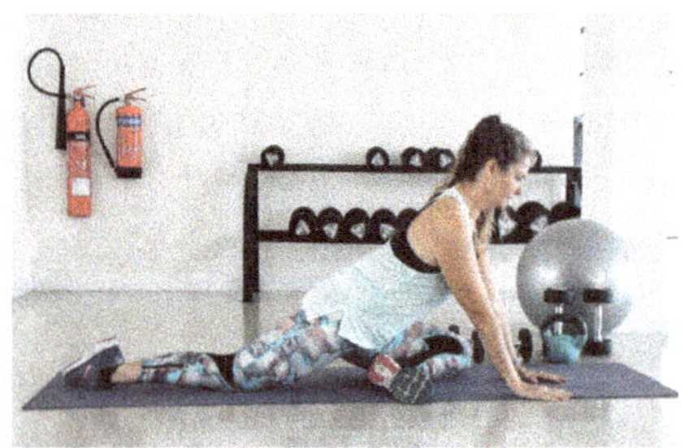

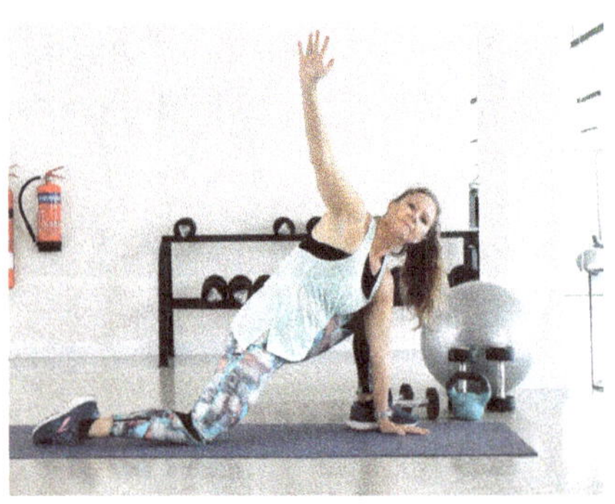

Next is a **GLUTE STRETCH**. Lie flat on your back and bend both knees. Cross one leg over the other so your foot is on the opposite knee.

Action: Bring both knees towards your chest and gently pull the uncrossed leg towards you until you feel a stretch in your buttock. Hold for 30 secs - like a pretzel!

HAMSTRING STRETCHING is really important, don't just focus on the front..

The right leg should be straight with a slight bend in the knee, and the bottom of the foot should face the ceiling. Gently pull with a strap or towel (if you need to) until there is a slight tension in the hamstrings. Hold the stretch for 10–30 seconds.

THORACIC OPENER - we all need this!

Stand with your feet hips-width distance apart. Interlace your hands behind your back and squeeze your shoulder blades together to stretch your chest.

If you have the mobility, keep your legs straight, bend at the hips, tucking your chin and bringing your hands over your head.

Relax the back of your neck, and if the stretch is too intense, release your hands, placing them on the backs of your thighs, and soften your knees. Hold for 20 to 30 seconds and slowly roll up to standing.

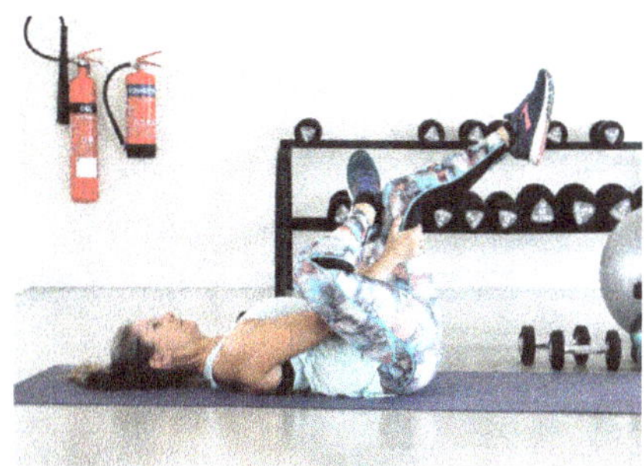

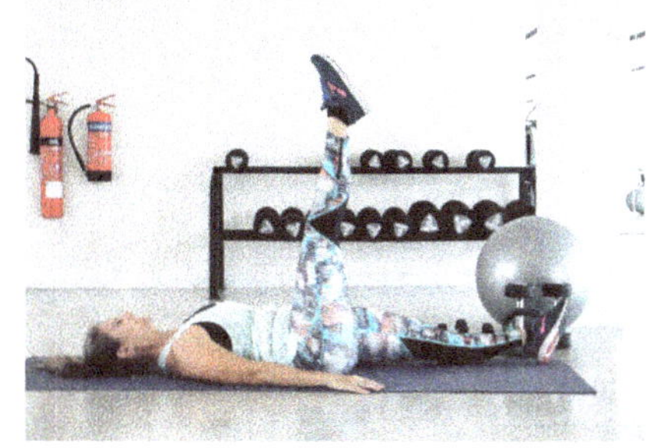

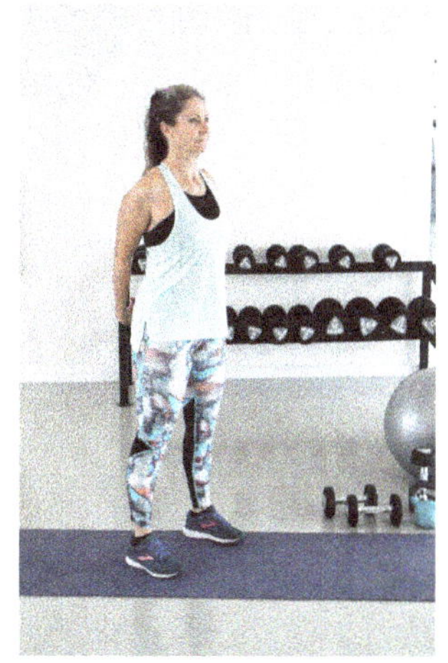

Now finish with a **DOWNWARD DOG** stretch. Begin in a kneeling position on your mat with hands directly under shoulders, fingers spread wide. Tuck your toes under and engage your abdominals as you push your body up off the mat so only your hands and feet are on the mat.

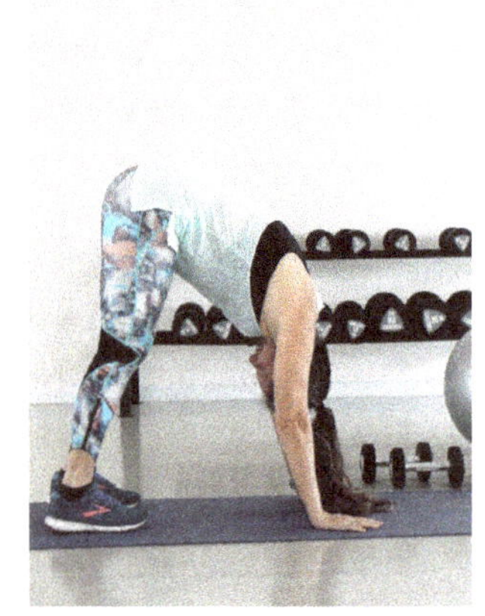

Press through your hands moving your chest gently toward your thighs and your heels gently toward the floor.

Relax your head and neck and breathe fully.

Abilities on this stretch will vary - don't panic! It will come.

Consistency is key!

So what's next?

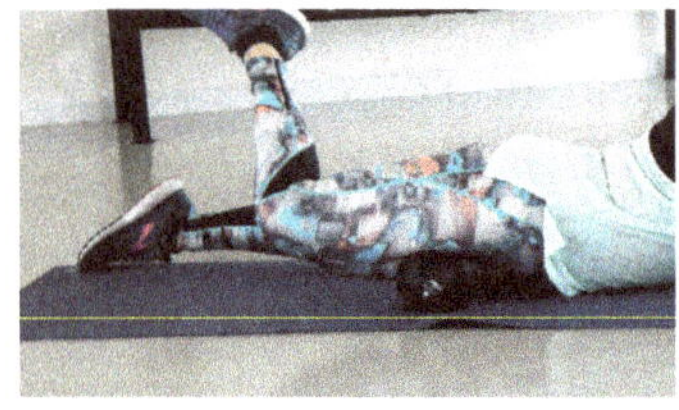

You've done all the training, you've been working out like a beast, but are you doing all the tissue care? It's time to get out the <u>roller</u> (again) and iron out your muscles. Stretch out your body and make sure that during the day, you get up from your chair and move. Do stuff like wall presses to encourage more mobility in your ankles, walk up the stairs at work and go see a colleague, spend 5 or 10 minutes moving your hips while you sip a hot beverage.

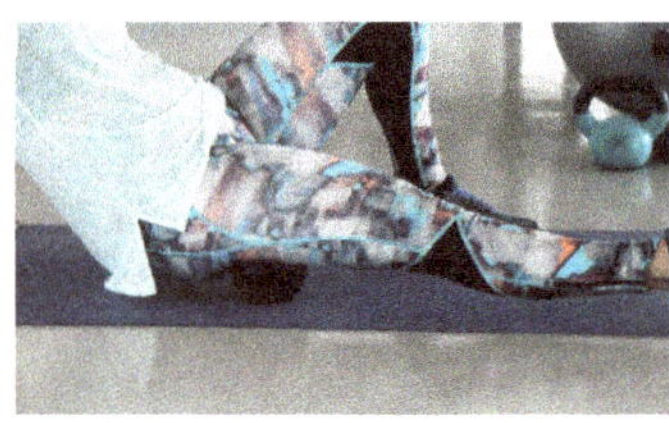

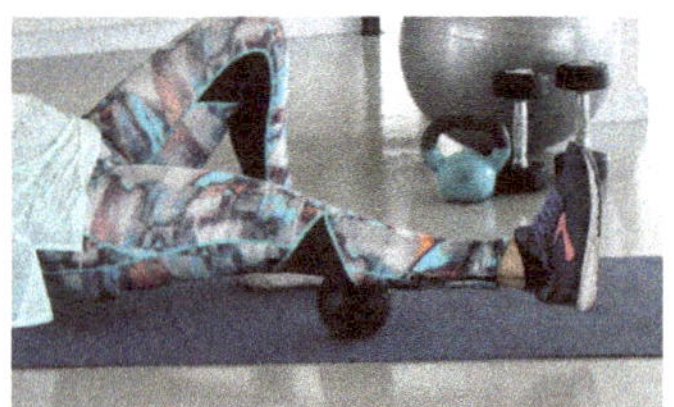

RECOVERY

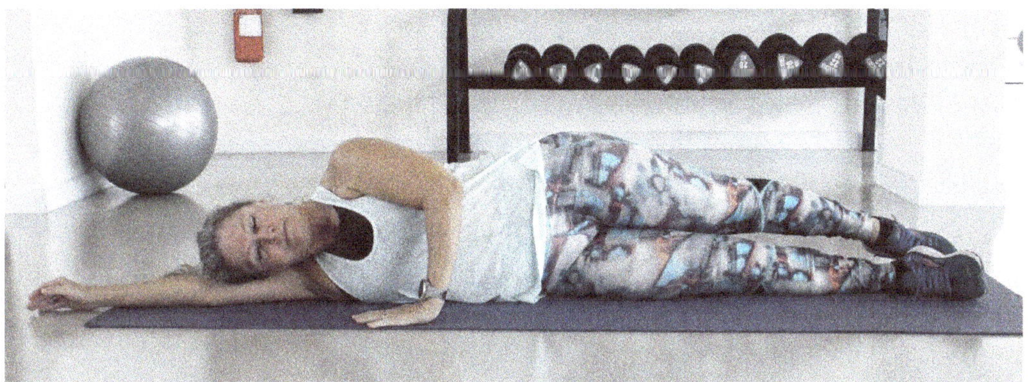

So what's next?

You've done all the training, you've been working out like a beast, but are you doing all the tissue care? It's time to get out the roller (again) and iron out your muscles. Stretch out your body and make sure that during the day, you get up from your chair and move. Do stuff like wall presses to encourage more mobility in your ankles, walk up the stairs at work and go see a colleague, spend 5 or 10 minutes moving your hips while you sip a beverage.

After your workouts you can follow this routine, available on YouTube. Check out my YouTube channel https://www.youtube.com/@saraharriscoaching1476

An important thing to note is that when it comes to SIT (or HIT), injuries are often due to overtraining. Overtraining occurs when there is too much volume or intensity (or both), and too little recovery time between exercise sessions. **AS A WOMAN IN MENOPAUSE, YOU MAY NOT RECOGNIZE OR BE ABLE TO DISTINGUISH IT AS THE SIGNS OF OVERTRAINING CAN MIMIC SIGNS OF MENOPAUSE.**

Monitor yourself and your recovery periods carefully. Speak to your physiotherapist or your sports doctor regularly and don't guess what's going on!

If you have any further questions regarding this guide, please do not hesitate to get in touch. I will happily reply!

HOW TO PLAN YOUR TRAINING

Many ask if they need to be spending 10 hours every week at the training helm. The short answer is NO and I can give you an achievable programme, whether it be to improve your body composition and lean up, or train for an endurance event.

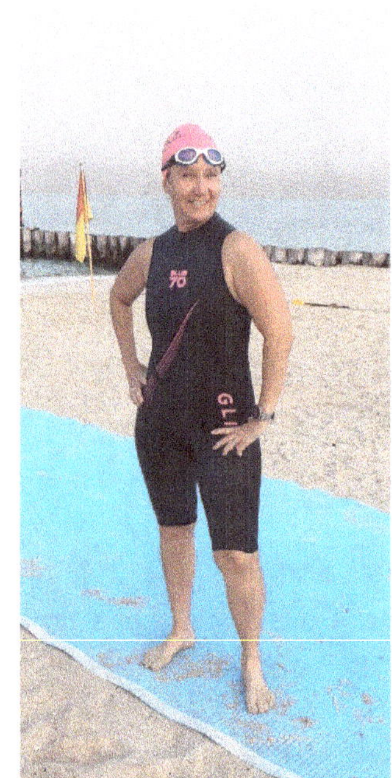

Like any new sport or even restarting training after illness, the most significant barrier you might experience is fear. I talk about fear a lot, as I have experienced it in the past, and the worst kind. Fear can break down your confidence, cause an unnecessary wobbly, shatter your belief in being able to finish, or start! If you can, training with a tribe can really help you with your fears and boost your confidence immensely. If you don't have a tribe, have a look on the internet in your area. There's got to be a group of people in a similar boat.

We all started at zero, at some point!

Can't Stop, Won't Stop

A training plan is essential to structured, accurate and efficient training. How have you programmed your weekly training sessions?

Are you trying to hit it hard in every session?

Are you doing two hard weeks, followed by an easier week? What is the split of your disciplines and the effort level in each?

If you are doing only strength training now, then you can do 5-6 sessions a week, and include one session with just mobility, and at least two (if not before and after every session) of rolling, hip openers, lateral lunges, single leg Bulgarian squats with overhead broomstick (rotate, too), glute bridges and rotational glute bridges.

Each strength session need only be 30-45 minutes.

CAPTURE YOUR JOURNEY

Now that you are motivated to start training, you can start journalling your training. Get a diary, or planner, or an excel spreadsheet, or even online software such as Training Peaks or Trainer Road, and mark out your training days, and what you will do with those days.

If you create a training schedule, you are more likely to stick to it rather than just "going down the gym" every day without a purpose. Mix your training up with some cross training, like swimming (go for lessons?), or getting out on your bike, going for a hike, run the dog on beach etc. Then programme your next day as a rest day or something light, like a swim to relax. Whichever way you choose, make sure it suits YOU, your needs, your body, and your goals. The journey is entirely your own. Claim it.

For example:

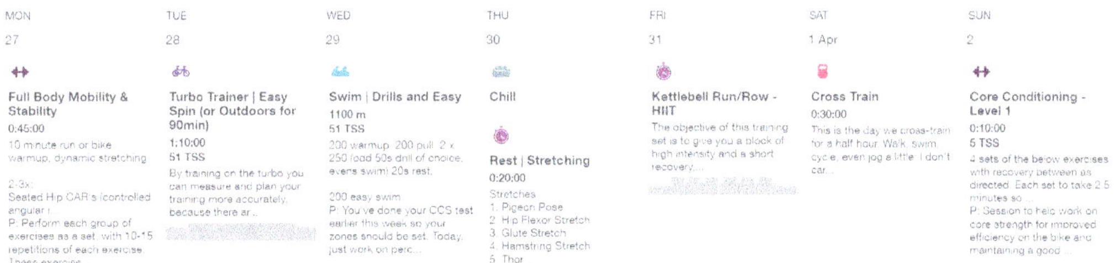

Day 1 - Game on - with a whole body workout for 45 minutes or mobility with core.

Day 2 - Easy spin on your bike to continue the week in a good mood.

Day 3 - Start the day with a swim, either at the pool or wild swimming if it's possible. Try to swim at least a kilometre.

Day 4 - Chill out, stretching, and always put in some mobility.

Day 5 - Now get on to a kettlebell routine, a good HIIT session (or SIT).

Day 6 - Cross Train - so here you could get on the elliptical with a podcast, treadmill if the weather is inclement, the rowing machine (excellent!) or again, out on your bike with friends - easy pace, low heart rate.

Day 7 - Do a Core routine - need only be 10 -20 minutes (See what I did there, hard-hard-easy, rest, hard-hard-easy).

The primary goal of any training programme is to prepare you for a specific event or outcome. Your journey will be different to every other person attempting the same programme. Individual requirements of frequency, volume, and intensity of training are different for each female athlete, and an imbalance between training-induced fatigue and recovery can manifest in various ways.

In my programmes I have considered that some women suffer excess fatigue or overtraining syndromes, while others seem to be able to go forever. If needed, you can pare back or increase the training frequency of each of your disciplines by about 10% if you feel either way. The idea is to gain improvements in fitness capacities and performance, while avoiding setbacks. Practice, make notes, detail your journey so you can understand what you did, how, and if you need or can afford more intensity, or even pull back a bit.

Be aware there can be setbacks in training and can include injury and/or illness due to improper nutrition, poor recovery and even psychological impairments. Consistency in your training, nutrition, hydration, and sleep will be key to avoiding these.

If you experience any of these symptoms, especially from a physiological standpoint please consult with your doctor and make sure that you are not exposing yourself to any possible side-effects (Low Energy Availability being a very common athletic ailment).

REFERENCES

Comparison of Strength-Training Adaptations in Early and Older Postmenopausal Women Rosario, Eric Joseph;Villani, Rudolph Gino;Harris, Jeff;Klein, Rudi Less

The effects of exercise and hormone replacement on muscle mass and strength (Changes in muscle mass and strength after menopause M.L. Maltais, J. Desroches, I.J. Dionne)

The Efficacy of Strength Exercises for Reducing the Symptoms of Menopause: A Systematic Review Ana María Capel-Alcaraz Héctor García-López, Adelaida María Castro-Sánchez, Manuel Fernández-Sánchez and Inmaculada Carmen Lara-Palomo

The Effect of Sprint Interval Training on Body Composition of Postmenopausal Women Yati N Boutcher Stephen H Boutcher Hye Y Yoo Jarrod D Meerkin

Effects of resistance training and detraining on muscle strength and blood lipid profiles in postmenopausal women. K J Elliott, C Sale, T Cable

Dupuit, Marine, Rance, Melanie, Morel, Claire, Bouillon, Patrice, Pereira, Bruno, Bonnet, Alban, et al. (2020). Moderate-Intensity Continuous Training or High-Intensity Interval Training with or without Resistance Training for Altering Body Composition in Postmenopausal Women. Medicine & Science in Sports & Exercise, 52, 736-745.

Eckert, Ryan & Snarr, Ronald. (2016). Kettlebell Training: A Brief Review. Journal of Sport and Human Performance. 4. 1-10

A hierarchical model of intrinsic and extrinsic motivation for sport and physical activity. Vallerand,

R. J. (2007)

Effects of single- vs. Multiple-set resistance training on maximum strength and body composition in trained postmenopausal women. Kemmler, Wolfgang K.1; Lauber, Dirk2; Engelke, Klaus1; Weineck, Juergen

The exercise-induced growth hormone response in athletes Richard J Godfrey 1, Zahra Madgwick,

Gregory P Whyte https://www.frontiersin.org/articles/10.3389/fphys.2018.01834/full

https://www.ncbi.nlm.nih.gov/pubmed/7484276/, https://www.ncbi.nlm.nih.gov/pubmed/11782642/ Resistance training: Shaw, Brandon S.; Gouveia, Monique; McIntyre, Shannon; Shaw, Ina. Anthropometric and cardiovascular responses to hypertrophic resistance training in postmenopausal women. Menopause, Volume 23, Number 11, November 2016, pp. 1176-1181(6).

The effects of hormone replacement therapy and resistance training on spine bone mineral density in early postmenopausal women Gianni F. Maddalozzo a, Jeffrey J. Widrick a, Bradley J. Cardinal a, Kerri M. Winters-Stone b, Mark A. Hoffman a, Christine M. Snow

Plyometric training: Vetrovsky, T., Steffl, M., Stastny, P. et al. The Efficacy and Safety of Lower-Limb Plyometric Training in Older Adults: A Systematic Review. Sports Med 49, 113–131 (2019).

Weight Lifted in Strength Training Predicts Bone Change in Postmenopausal Women Ellen c. Cussler, Timothy G. Lohman, Scott B. Going Linda B. Houtkooper, Lauve L. Metcalfe, Hilary g. Flint- wagner, Robin B. Harris, and Pedro J. Teixeira

Metabolic Syndrome: Updates on Pathophysiology and Management in 2021 Gracia Fahed, Laurence Aoun, Morgan Bou Zerdan, Sabine Allam, Maroun Bou Zerdan, Youssef Bouferraa, and Hazem I. Assi

Exercise and the growth hormone-insulin-like growth factor axis Jan Frystyk

Effects of Kettlebell Load on Joint Kinetics and Global Characteristics during Overhead Swings in Women Cullun Q. Watts, Kirsten Boessneck and Bryan L. Riemann

The Effect of Kettlebell Swing Load and Cadence on Physiological, Perceptual and Mechanical Variables Michael J. Duncan Rosanna Gibbard Leanne M. Raymond Peter Mundy

Kettlebell Research Update Len Kravitz, Ph.D

Cardiovascular and Metabolic Demands of the Kettlebell Swing using Tabata Interval versus a Traditional Resistance Protocol HOWARD A. FORTNER, JEANETTE M. SALGADO ANGELICA M. HOLMSTRUP, and MICHAEL E. HOLMSTRUP

Coaching effectiveness: Exploring the relationship between coaching behavior and self-determined motivation. Ryan & Deci, 2007.

Dr Stacy Sims - Next Level Dr Stacy Sims - ROAR Feisty Menopause

NESTA - Kettlebell Coach Programme 2019

Manual of Structural Kinesiology R.T. Floyd, EdD, ATC, CSCS https://www.kettlebellkings.com/

Research into the Health Benefits of Sprint Interval Training Should Focus on Protocols with Fewer and Shorter Sprints Niels B J Vollaard 1, Richard S Metcalfe

Menopause: Highlighting the Effects of Resistance Training R. D. Leite1, J. Prestes, G. B. Pereira, G. E. Shiguemoto, S. E. A. Perez

Phil Mosley, Triathlon Coach

www.ingramcontent.com/pod-product-compliance
Lightning Source LLC
Chambersburg PA
CBHW080915160726
48000CB00009B/3001